BLUEPRINTS
RADIOLOGY

Second Edition

For every step of your medical career, look for all the books in the *Blueprints* series

Perfect for clerkship and board review!

Blueprints Cardiology, 2nd edition
Blueprints Emergency Medicine, 2nd edition
Blueprints Family Medicine, 2nd edition
Blueprints Medicine, 3rd edition
Blueprints Neurology, 2nd edition
Blueprints Obstetrics & Gynecology, 3rd edition
Blueprints Pediatrics, 3rd edition
Blueprints Psychiatry, 3rd edition
Blueprints Radiology, 2nd edition
Blueprints Surgery, 3rd edition

Visit www.blackwellmedstudent.com to see all the great *Blueprints*:

Blueprints Notes & Cases
Blueprints Clinical Cases
Blueprints Pockets
Blueprints Step 2 Q&A
Blueprints USMLE Step 2 CS
Blueprints Step 3 Q&A
Blueprints Computer-Based Case Simulation Review: USMLE Step 3
Blueprints Clinical Procedures

BLUEPRINTS
RADIOLOGY

Second Edition

Alina Uzelac, DO
Resident, Department of Radiology
Los Angeles County/
University of Southern California Medical Center
Los Angeles, California

Ryan W. Davis, MD
MRI Fellow, Department of Radiology
University of Southern California Medical Center
Los Angeles, California

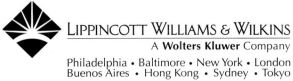

LIPPINCOTT WILLIAMS & WILKINS
A **Wolters Kluwer** Company

Philadelphia • Baltimore • New York • London
Buenos Aires • Hong Kong • Sydney • Tokyo

Acquisitions Editor: Beverly Copland
Development Editor: Kate Heinle
Production Editor: Debra Murphy
Cover and Interior Designer: Mary McKeon
Compositor: TechBooks in New Delhi, India
Printer: Walsworth Publishing in Marceline, MO

Copyright © 2006 Alina Uzelac, DO

351 West Camden Street
Baltimore, MD 21201

530 Walnut Street
Philadelphia, PA 19106

The publisher is not responsible (as a matter of product liability, negligence, or otherwise) for any injury resulting from any material contained herein. This publication contains information relating to general principles of medical care that should not be construed as specific instructions for individual patients. Manufacturers' product information and package inserts should be reviewed for current information, including contraindications, dosages, and precautions.

Printed in the United States of America

Library of Congress Cataloging-in-Publication Data

Uzelac, Alina.
    Blueprints radiology / Alina Uzelac, Ryan W. Davis. — 2nd ed.
      p. ; cm. — (Blueprints series)
    Rev. ed. of: Blueprints in radiology / by Ryan W. Davis, Mitchell
S. Komaiko, Barry D. Pressman. c2002.
    Includes index.
    ISBN-13: 978-1-4051-0460-9 (pbk. : alk. paper)
    ISBN-10: 1-4051-0460-0 (pbk. : alk. paper)
    1. Radiography, Medical—Outlines, syllabi, etc. 2. Radiography,
Medical—Examinations, questions, etc. I. Davis, Ryan W.
II. Davis, Ryan W. Blueprints in radiology. III. Title. IV. Title:
Radiology. V. Series: Blueprints.
    [DNLM: 1. Diagnostic Imaging—methods—Examination
Questions. 2. Radiography—methods—Examination Questions.
WN 18.2 U99b 2006]
RC78.17D385 2006
616.07'572'076—dc22

                          2005013092

The publishers have made every effort to trace the copyright holders for borrowed material. If they have inadvertently overlooked any, they will be pleased to make the necessary arrangements at the first opportunity.

To purchase additional copies of this book, call our customer service department at **(800) 638-3030** or fax orders to **(301) 824-7390**. International customers should call **(301) 714-2324**.

Visit Lippincott Williams & Wilkins on the Internet: *http://www.LWW.com.* Lippincott Williams & Wilkins customer service representatives are available from 8:30 am to 6:00 pm, EST.

                                   06 07 08 09
                           2 3 4 5 6 7 8 9 10

Table of Contents

Contributors

Andrei H. Iagaru, MD
Resident, Division of Nuclear Medicine
Los Angeles County/
University of Southern California Medical Center
Clinical Instructor
Keck School of Medicine
University of Southern California
Los Angeles, California

Sam K. Kim, MD
Resident, Department of Radiology
Los Angeles County/
University of Southern California Medical Center
Los Angeles, California

Reviewers

Kenneth Bryant, PhD, MD
Resident, Radiology Department
University of Texas Houston
Houston, Texas

Aimee P. Carswell, MD
Intern
University of Texas Health Science Center at San Antonio
San Antonio, Texas

James Chen, MD
Resident, Radiology Department
University of California San Francisco
San Francisco, California

Celeste Chu-Kuo, MD
Resident, Pediatrics
Saint Louis Children's Hospital
St. Louis, Missouri

Danielle Fournier
Class of 2005
Northeastern University PA Program
Boston, Massachusetts

Scott M. Greenberg, DO
Resident, Orthopedic Surgery
Palmetto General Hospital
Miami, Florida

Deneta Howland, MD
Resident, Department of Pediatrics
Morehouse School of Medicine
Atlanta, Georgia

Kimmy Jong
Class of 2005
Loma Linda University School of Medicine
Loma Linda, California

Brent Luria
Class of 2005
McGill University
Montreal, Quebec
Canada

Susan Merel
Class of 2005
Pritzker School of Medicine
University of Chicago
Chicago, Illinois

Azam Mohiuddin
Class of 2005
University of Kentucky College of Medicine
Lexington, Kentucky

Ai Mukai, MD
Preliminary Medicine Resident
Pennsylvania State College of Medicine
Hershey, Pennsylvania

Mark A. Naftanel
Class of 2005
Duke University School of Medicine
Durham, North Carolina

David E. Ruchelsman
Class of 2004
New York University School of Medicine
New York, New York

Tina Small
Class of 2005
Quinnipiac University PA Program
Hamden, Connecticut

Christopher J. Steen, MD
Intern, Transitional Program
Saint Barnabas Medical Center
Livingston, New Jersey

Jacqui Thomas
Class of 2005
Nova Southeastern University
Miami, Florida

Abraham Tzou, MD
Resident, Department of Laboratory Medicine
Yale University School of Medicine
New Haven, Connecticut

Debra Zynger
Class of 2004
Indiana University School of Medicine
Indianapolis, Indiana

Preface

In 1997, the first five books in the **Blueprints** series were published as board review for medical students, interns, and residents who wanted high-yield, accurate clinical content for USMLE Steps 2 & 3. Nearly a decade later, the **Blueprints** brand has expanded into high-quality, trusted resources covering the broad range of clinical topics studied by medical students and residents during their primary, specialty, and subspecialty rotations.

The **Blueprints** were conceived as a study aid created by students, for students. In keeping with this concept, the editors of the current edition of the **Blueprints** books have recruited resident contributors to ensure that the series continues to offer the information and the approach that made the original **Blueprints** a success.

Now in their second edition, each of the five specialty **Blueprints**—**Blueprints** *Emergency Medicine*, **Blueprints** *Family Medicine*, **Blueprints** *Neurology*, **Blueprints** *Cardiology*, and **Blueprints** *Radiology*—has been completely revised and updated to bring you the most current treatment and management strategies. The feedback we have received from our readers has been tremendously helpful in guiding the editorial direction of the second edition. We are grateful to the hundreds of medical students and residents who have responded with in-depth comments and highly detailed observations.

Each book has been thoroughly reviewed and revised accordingly, with new features included across the series. An evidence-based resource section has been added to provide current and classic references for each chapter, and an increased number of current board-format questions with detailed explanations for correct and incorrect answer options is included in each book. All revisions to the **Blueprints** series have been made in order to offer you the most concise, comprehensive, and cost-effective information available.

Our readers report that **Blueprints** are useful for every step of their medical career—from their clerkship rotations and subinternships to a board review for USMLE Steps 2 & 3. Residents studying for USMLE Step 3 often use the books for reviewing areas that were not their specialty. Students from a wide variety of health care specialties, including those in physician assistant, nurse practitioner, and osteopathic programs, use **Blueprints** either as a course companion or to review for their licensure examinations.

However you use **Blueprints**, we hope you find the books in the series informative and useful. Your feedback and suggestions are essential to our continued success. Please send any comments you may have about this or any book in the **Blueprints** series to medfeedback@bos.blackwellpublishing.com.

Thank you for your willingness to share your opinions, offer constructive feedback, and to support our products.

The Publisher
Blackwell Publishing, Inc.

Abbreviations

ABCDE	(approach) air, bones, cardiac, diaphragm, everything else
ABI	ankle-brachial index
ACA	anterior cerebral artery
ACE	angiotensin-converting enzyme
AIDS	acquired immunodeficiency syndrome
AP	anterior-posterior
ARDS	adult respiratory distress syndrome
BUN	blood urea nitrogen
CAD	coronary artery disease
CBC	complete blood cell (count)
COPD	chronic obstructive pulmonary disease
CSF	cerebrospinal fluid
CT	computed tomography
CTPA	computed tomography pulmonary angiography
CXR	chest x-ray
DISIDA	di-isopropyl iminodiacetic acid
DVT	deep vein thrombosis
DWI	diffusion-weighted imaging
ECG	electrocardiogram
EEC	endometrial echo complex
EEG	electroencephalogram
ESR	erythrocyte sedimentation rate
GB	gallbladder
GCS	Glasgow Coma Score
GFR	glomerular filtration rate
GI	gastrointestinal
H_2	histamine-2
hCG	human chorionic gonadotropin
HIV	human immunodeficiency virus
HLA	human leukocyte antigen
HU	Hounsfield units
^{123}I	iodine-123
IgE	immunoglobulin E
IAC	internal auditory canal
INR	international normalized ratio
IV	intravenous
IVC	inferior vena cava
IVP	intravenous pyelogram
KUB	kidneys, ureters, bladder
LDH	lactate dehydrogenase
MAA	macroaggregated albumin
MACHINE	metabolic, autoimmune, congenital, hematologic, infectious, neoplastic, environmental
MCA	middle cerebral artery
MI	myocardial infarction
MMSE	Mini-Mental Status Examination
MRA	magnetic resonance angiography
MRCP	magnetic resonance cholangiopancreatography
MRI	magnetic resonance imaging
MRS	magnetic resonance spectroscopy
MUGA	multiple-gated angiography
MVA	motor-vehicle accident
NF	neurofibromatosis
NPO	nothing by mouth
PA	posterior-anterior
PCA	posterior cerebral artery
PE	pulmonary embolism
PET	positron emission tomography
PFA	profunda femoris artery
PIOPED	Prospective Investigation of Pulmonary Embolism Diagnosis
PMN	polymorphonuclear
PO	by mouth
PSA	prostate-specific antigen
PT	prothrombin time
PTA	percutaneous transluminal angioplasty
PTT	partial thromboplastin time
RBC	red blood cell (count)
RDS	respiratory distress syndrome
RF	radiofrequency
RPS	retropharyngeal space
SALTR	slipped, above, lower, through, ruined (Salter-Harris fracture types)
SGOT	serum glutamic oxaloacetic transaminase
SPECT	single-photon emission computed tomography

^{89}SR	strontium-89	TR	time to repeat
STD	sexually transmitted disease	UPJ	ureteropelvic junction
TB	tuberculosis	UVJ	ureterovesicular junction
^{99m}Tc	technetium-99m	VCUG	voiding cystourethrogram
TE	time to echo	V/Q	ventilation-perfusion
^{201}Tl	thallium-201	WBC	white blood cell (count)

Chapter 1

General Principles in Radiology

In 1895 Dutch physicist Wilhelm Roentgen discovered the x-ray, and since that time, many uses for it have been developed in both diagnostic and therapeutic medicine. The specialty of radiology includes conventional techniques that use ionizing radiation, such as radiography (plain film), fluoroscopy, computed tomography (CT), and nuclear medicine. It also includes the techniques of magnetic resonance imaging (MRI) and ultrasound, which produce images with magnetic fields and sound waves, respectively, thereby avoiding the risks of radiation.

■ RADIOGRAPHY AND FLUOROSCOPY

A standard x-ray machine (Figure 1-1) generates high-energy photons, or **x-rays,** as they are also called, with a high-voltage electric current. The x-rays are directed in a focused beam toward the patient. They then pass through the patient to the film; they are absorbed by the patient's tissues; or they scatter, in which case they will not provide diagnostic information. As the x-rays reach the cassette and interact with the radiographic film, their energy is converted into visible light, which exposes the film and creates the familiar radiograph. In fluoroscopy the film is replaced by an image intensifier, which allows a digital image to be seen on a television monitor in real time.

A radiograph is a two-dimensional representation of the three-dimensional structures of the patient's body. These structures are visible because of the differences in attenuation of the x-ray beam. **Attenuation** refers to the process by which x-rays are removed from the primary x-ray beam through absorption and scatter. Attenuated x-rays are essentially "blocked" and never reach the film to expose it. The degree of attenuation by the tissues of the body

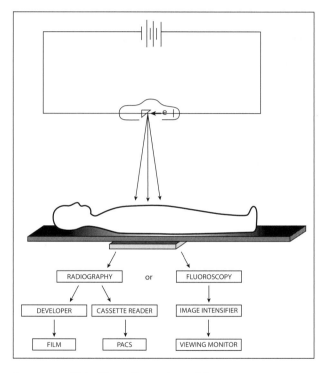

Figure 1-1 • Plain-film radiography and fluoroscopy.

is based on three main factors: tissue thickness in the line of the x-ray beam, the density of the tissue, and the atomic number of the material through which the beam passes (Table 1-1).

Unexposed film, which corresponds to high attenuation of the x-ray beam, appears bright on the radiograph, as with bone, for example. Exposed film, which corresponds to low attenuation of the x-ray beam, appears dark, as with air in the lungs. The terms **radiolucency** and **radiodensity** relate to attenuation along the same scale; air is the most radiolucent, and

■ TABLE 1-1

The Five Main Radiodensities on a Standard Radiograph

Material	Effective Atomic Number	Density (g/cm³)	Color on Film
Air	7.6	RADIOLUCENT 0.001	
Fat	5.9	0.9	
Water (Organ tissue, muscle skin, blood	7.4	1	
Bone	14.0	2	
Metal	82.0	RADIODENSE 11	

bone is the most radiodense. A gradient of gray, corresponding to all the remaining tissue types, lies between these two extremes. Four main tissue types are distinguished on a radiograph, and, in order of increasing attenuation, they are air, fat, soft tissue, and bone.

Distinctions between tissues can be made only when there is an interface with differences in density between the tissues. For instance, air bronchograms are evident in a lung segment with pneumonia because there is an interface between the air inside the bronchi and the pus-filled alveoli of the lung tissue. As a demonstration, a balloon filled with water is placed inside a glass, also filled with water (Figure 1-2). Because there is essentially a "water-water" interface with the thin membrane of the balloon between, the balloon is not seen on a radiograph. If the balloon is filled with air, an "air-water" interface is created, and the shape of the balloon becomes evident on the radiograph.

Plain radiographs are useful as first-line examinations of the chest, abdomen, and skeletal structures. Some common indications for chest radiographs are shortness of breath, chest pain, and cough. For abdominal plain films, common indications are abdominal pain, vomiting, and trauma. Skeletal films are useful in evaluating osseous trauma, arthritis, bone neoplasms, metabolic bone disease, and congenital dysplasias. The limitation of plain radiographs is due to the two-dimensional reproduction of three-dimensional structures; so often the location of the lesion cannot be established without using a more accurate localizing modality (e.g., CT, ultrasound, or MRI).

KEY POINTS

1. The familiar radiograph is a two-dimensional representation of the three-dimensional structures of the patient's body.
2. Four main tissue types are distinguished on a radiograph; in order of increasing attenuation, they are air, fat, soft tissue, and bone.
3. Distinctions between tissues can be made only when there is an interface with differences in density between the tissues.
4. Plain radiographs are useful as first-line examinations of the chest, abdomen, and skeletal structures.

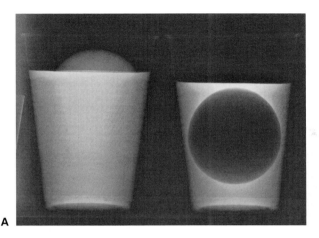

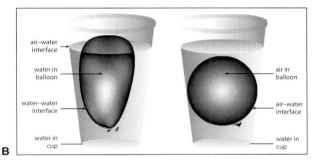

Figure 1-2 • A: Radiographic demonstration of interfaces. On the left, a balloon filled with water rests inside a cup filled with water. The "water-water" interface cannot be seen because there is no difference in attenuation. On the right, a balloon filled with air rests inside a cup filled with water. An "air-water" interface is demonstrated and the air appears black inside the water, which is white. (Courtesy of Cedars-Sinai Medical Center, Los Angeles, CA.) **B:** Diagrammatic representation of the radiographic interfaces in (A).

IMAGING MODALITIES

▇ COMPUTED TOMOGRAPHY

Computed tomography (CT) is a method of using x-rays in multiple projections to produce axial images of the body. The image production differs from conventional radiography in that the x-rays pass through the patient to highly sensitive detectors instead of film. These detectors then send the information to a computer that reconstructs the images (Figure 1-3). The images are displayed in an anatomic position as if one is observing the patient while standing at the feet and looking toward the head. Any body part can

be imaged, but generally examinations are divided into head, neck, spine, chest, abdomen, pelvis, and extremities. The patient lies supine on the examination table, which moves horizontally through the frame, or **gantry,** as it is commonly called.

In CT, adjacent anatomic structures are delineated by the differences in attenuation between them. Again, **attenuation** refers to the physical properties of the molecules in the body that contribute to absorption and scatter of the x-ray beams. These properties differentially prevent some x-rays from reaching the detectors on the opposite side of the gantry.

CT is more sensitive than conventional plain film in distinguishing differences of tissue density, which are displayed in Hounsfield units (HU) in a range of approximately (-1000) to $(+1000)$, corresponding to a gradient scale of gray. Generally one can divide densities for CT into seven categories (with their HU ranges) (Table 1-2).

Two important concepts arise in discussion of the HU gray scale: "window" and "level." **Window** refers to the range across which the computer will display the shades of gray on the monitor for viewing. A narrow window produces greater contrast. **Level** is the midpoint value in HUs of the scale and is used to view preferentially the different types of tissue. For

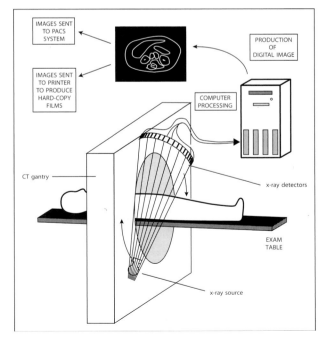

Figure 1-3 • Standard CT system and production of axial CT images.

TABLE 1-2

Housenfield Units on CT

CT into seven general categories (with their HU ranges):

1. Air (−1000 to −200 HU)

2. Fat (−50 to 0 HU)

3. Water (0 to 10 HU)

4. Soft tissue (20 to 50 HU)

5. Non-flowing blood (50 to 70 HU)

6. Bone (+300 to −500 HU)

7. Metal (+500 to +1000 HU)

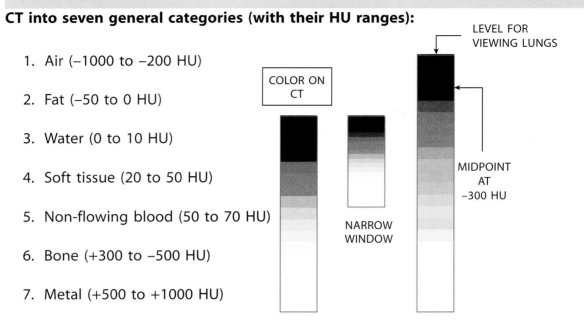

example, to examine lung detail, one would choose a low value (−300 HU) for the level instead of the higher HU values of soft tissue and bone.

Common uses of CT include examining any part of the body where fine anatomic detail or subtle distinction between tissue types is necessary for diagnosis. Examples include a head CT to exclude bleeding or a skull fracture in head trauma, a chest CT to evaluate nodules or masses, an abdominal CT for metastatic workup or in the presence of fever of unknown origin to exclude abscess, and a skeletal CT to evaluate subtle fractures not clearly seen on plain films.

No modality is perfect, and CT has its limitations. At times a liver carcinoma may not be conspicuous on CT but can be seen only on MRI. An aortic laceration or a small pulmonary embolus can sometimes be detected only by conventional angiogram, and a negative CT is not sufficient to exclude the presence of either.

NUCLEAR MEDICINE

Nuclear medicine differs from conventional radiography in several fundamental ways. First, rather than delivering x-rays externally through the patient to produce an image, a dose of radiation is given internally to the patient and the x-rays are counted

KEY POINTS

1. CT is a method of using x-rays to produce axial images of the body; these images are viewed as if looking from the feet up toward the head.
2. CT is more sensitive than conventional plain film in distinguishing differences of tissue density.
3. Common uses of CT include examining any part of the body where fine anatomic detail or subtle distinction between tissue types is necessary for diagnosis.

as they leave his or her body. Second, some nuclear medicine studies provide functional information in addition to the anatomic information of conventional radiographic techniques. The radiation dose or radionuclide is usually given either orally (PO) or intravenously (IV), and it has an affinity for certain organs. As the radionuclide decays, it emits gamma radiation, which is detected by special cameras that count the number of emitted photons and send the information to a computer (Figure 1-4). The computer processes the data with regard to the source location and the number of counts to form an image or series of images over time.

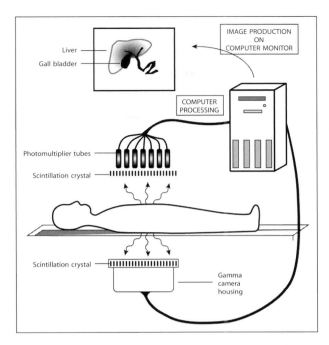

Figure 1-4 • Standard two-head gamma camera and production of nuclear medicine scintigraphy images.

Common uses of nuclear medicine studies are ventilation-perfusion (V/Q) scan for suspected pulmonary embolism; di-isopropyl iminodiacetic acid (DISIDA) scan for suspected acute cholecystitis; bone scan or positron emission tomography (PET) for metastatic workup; diethylenetriamine pentaacetic acid (DTPA) renal scan for renal failure; gallium scan for lymphoma or occult infection; indium-tagged white blood cell scan for occult infection; iodine-123 (^{123}I) scan for thyroid nodules; and technetium-tagged red blood cell (RBC) scan for gastrointestinal (GI) bleeding and hepatic hemangioma evaluation.

The most important limitation of nuclear medicine studies is their decreased spatial resolution.

KEY POINTS

1. In nuclear medicine studies, a dose of radiation is given internally to the patient and the x-rays are counted as they leave his or her body.
2. Some nuclear medicine studies provide functional information in addition to the anatomic information of conventional radiographic techniques.

ULTRASOUND

In ultrasonography, a probe is applied to the patient's skin, and a high frequency (1 to 20 MHz) beam of sound waves is focused on the area of interest (Figure 1-5). The sound waves propagate through different tissues at different velocities, with denser tissues allowing the sound waves to move faster. A detector measures the time it takes for the wave to reflect and return to the probe. Tissue density is determined by the reflection time, and an image is produced on the screen for the ultrasonographer to see in real time.

Normal soft tissue appears as medium **echogenicity,** the term for brightness on ultrasound. Fat is usually more echogenic than soft tissue is. Simple fluid, such as bile, has low echogenicity, appears dark, and often has "through-transmission," or brightness beyond it. Complex fluid, such as blood or pus, may have strands or septations within it, and it generally has lower through-transmission than does simple fluid. Calcification usually appears as high echogenicity with posterior "shadowing," or a dark "band" beyond it. Air does not transmit sound waves well and does not permit imaging beyond it; the sound waves do not reflect back to the transducer. Therefore, bowel gas and lung tissue are hindrances to ultrasound imaging.

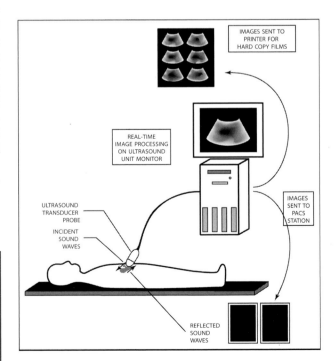

Figure 1-5 • Standard ultrasound system and production of ultrasonographic images.

Common uses of ultrasound include evaluating the gallbladder for suspected cholecystitis, the pancreas for pancreatitis, and the right lower quadrant of the abdomen in suspected appendicitis. Other indications include evaluation of the liver, pancreas, or kidneys for masses or evidence of obstruction. Ultrasound is also very helpful in the evaluation of pelvic pain in women and in suspected ectopic pregnancy, ovarian torsion, or pelvic masses. Finally, with the use of Doppler imaging in ultrasonography, which detects flow velocity and direction, one can image blood vessels such as the aorta for suspected aneurysm, and the deep leg veins or portal vein for thrombosis.

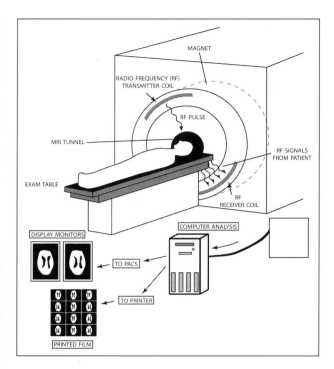

Figure 1-6 • Standard MRI magnet and production of MR images.

KEY POINTS

1. Ultrasound imaging uses the reflection of high-frequency sound waves to generate images of the patient's internal organs.
2. Bowel gas and lung tissue are a hindrance to ultrasound imaging.
3. Common uses of ultrasound include evaluating the gallbladder, pancreas, liver, and kidneys for various pathologic conditions. Ultrasound is also useful in assessing acute pelvic pain in women and various other pathologic conditions of the pelvic organs.

■ MAGNETIC RESONANCE IMAGING

In general terms, MRI utilizes the physical principle that hydrogen protons will align when placed within a strong magnetic field. To obtain an MRI scan, the patient lies on the table within the scanner tube and is surrounded by a high-intensity magnetic field (Figure 1-6). Protons in the patient's tissues align with the vector of the magnetic field and a radiofrequency (RF) pulse is emitted from the transmitter coils, causing the protons to "deflect" perpendicular to their original vector. When the RF pulse ceases, the protons "relax" back to their original position, releasing energy, which is detected by the receiver coils of the scanner. The patient's tissues will generate different signals, depending on the relative hydrogen proton composition. These signals are processed by a computer to produce the final image.

T1 (short TR, short TE) sequence is useful for visualizing anatomic details (knee menisci tears, subacute hemorrhage, and fat [both these latter two are

bright on this sequence]). High-protein-content structures show high signal intensity on this sequence. The T1 sequence has limited delineation of edema- and water-containing pathology. This is the sequence used with gadolinium for enhancement of lesions and is great for demonstrating anatomy.

Structures with a high water content (including tumor, infection, injury) have high signal intensity on T2 (long TR and long TE) sequence (Figure 1-7).

Fat saturation techniques are very useful because they suppress the fat signal without affecting the water signal, and they make lesions stand out (i.e., they help to distinguish between fat and hemorrhage). Gradient echo sequence is used for its sensitivity for susceptibility artifacts (i.e., it detects small areas of hemorrhage resulting from hemoglobin breakdown products; soft-tissue gas; metallic particles, which cause a "blooming" artifact). All MRI sequences have advantages and drawbacks; therefore, for a high-quality study, an appropriate protocol must be created based on a clinical history and suspected pathology.

Magnetic resonance imaging has several advantages over CT. First, MRI does not use ionizing radiation and therefore avoids its potential harmful effects.

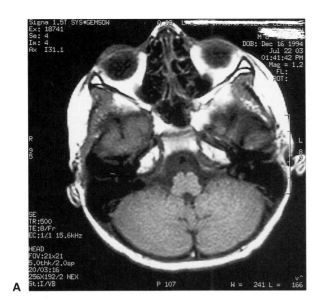 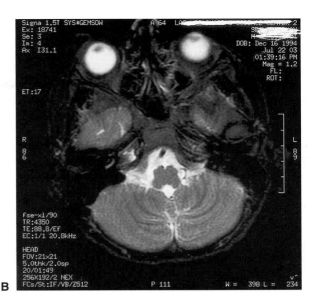

Figure 1-7 • Demonstration of T1- versus T2-weighted images. (A) On the T1 sequence, the fat is bright and the ocular globes and CSF (water) are dark, in contrast to T2 (B) (water is bright on T2s; see the CSF around the medulla oblongata and the vitreous of the ocular globes).
(Courtesy of University of Southern California Medical Center, Los Angeles, CA.)

Second, images can be easily obtained in any plane rather than only in the transverse plane, as with CT. Finally, MRI generally provides better anatomic detail of soft tissues and is better at detecting subtle pathologic differences. The disadvantages are that MRI takes much longer to scan a patient than CT; it is more expensive; and it has more contraindications, such as pacemakers, old material aneurysm clips, and metallic foreign bodies (i.e., intraocular), all of which can be adversely affected by the magnetic field. Magnetic resonance angiogram (MRA) for pulmonary embolus detection should be considered an alternative for pregnant patients, although small subsegmental pulmonary artery branch emboli will not be visualized.

Also, MRA can be used for aortic dissection (chronic, nonemergent type) or aneurysms.

CONTRAST MATERIAL

Contrast material increases the differences in density between anatomic structures. Gastrointestinal contrast agents such as barium and Gastrografin are used to outline the entire gastrointestinal tract for CT and fluoroscopic examinations. Oral contrast administration is seldom detrimental to the patient. However, there are particular instances in which administration of oral contrast should be restricted, such as in patients on strict nothing by mouth (NPO) status because of acute pancreatitis and in patients at risk for aspiration that would lead to a Gastrografin-induced pneumonitis. Aspirated barium is inert and is not damaging to the lung parenchyma. By contrast, if an esophageal perforation is expected, Gastrografin should be used instead of barium because barium is thought to cause mediastinitis. A suspected bowel perforation does not preclude use of Gastrografin because this agent will not cause peritonitis or affect the surgical field.

Intravenous contrast agents, such as iodine-based contrast for CT and gadolinium for MRI, are used to visualize vascular structures and to provide enhance-

---

KEY POINTS

1. MRI utilizes the physical principle that hydrogen protons will align when placed within a strong magnetic field.
2. The patient's tissues will generate different signals for the final MR image, depending on relative hydrogen proton composition.
3. MRI does not use ionizing radiation.
4. MRI generally provides better anatomic detail of soft tissues than does CT.

ment of organs. Gadolinium also helps to distinguish between cystic versus cystic-appearing lesions, a distinction that is sometimes difficult on MRI. This contrast agent can also be used intra-articularly for the detection of subtle joint or cartilaginous pathology.

Intravenous iodine-based contrast is seen within blood vessels, allowing them to be distinguished from lymph nodes and other soft-tissue structures of similar anatomic dimensions. It is therefore seen preferentially in areas of relatively high blood flow, identifying tumors, abscesses, or areas of inflammation. Contrast passes through leaky vascular spaces in tumors, increasing the attenuation of the tissue and making it more conspicuous. Iodine-based contrast also frequently yields a diagnosis based on its absence. For example, a filling defect within a blood vessel or solid organ likely indicates thrombus, hypoperfusion, or infarct.

Intravenous iodine-based contrast is mandatory for a chest CT if pulmonary embolism is suspected. Other uses include suspected solid-organ tumor to look for enhancement. If an abscess is suspected, contrast is helpful to delineate the margins of an infected cavity because of the relative hyperemia in the abscess walls, which appear as high attenuation on a CT scan.

The risks and benefits of IV iodine-based contrast should be considered before using it for a patient who has any renal compromise because of the risk of causing acute renal failure. IV iodine-based contrast is usually not given if the patient's creatinine level is greater than 1.5 unless the study is absolutely necessary. In cases of severe trauma, the creatinine levels are not drawn before the CT scan because time is crucial. An example would be in a case of trauma with suspected vascular, renal, or ureteral injury. If a patient is on dialysis, the iodinated contrast is cleared from the bloodstream by this treatment. In cases of renal insufficiency without overt failure, N-acetylcysteine (Mucomyst) 600 mg administered PO twice daily, preferably started 24 hours before the examination, is administered for a total of 72 hours. Concomitant good hydration is even more important because studies on the efficacy of this agent have not had as favorable results as previously thought, but it is currently the only treatment that attempts renal protection.

The contrast also carries a risk of causing allergic reactions, including anaphylaxis; however, allergic reactions are significantly less common with the newer nonionic contrast agents. Patients with a history of clinically significant allergic reaction to iodine should still be premedicated with diphenhydramine hydrochloride, prednisone, and a histamine 2 (H_2)-blocker such as cimetidine or ranitidine. If IV iodine contrast is to be given to a patient who uses the antidiabetic medication metformin, the medication must not be given for the subsequent 48 hours because of the risk of metabolic acidosis.

Iodinated contrast is used also in the fluoroscopically guided intravascular invasive procedures. Alternate contrast agents for patients with renal insufficiency or absolute contraindications to iodine are CO_2 gas or gadolinium, but the images are of limited quality.

KEY POINTS

1. Contrast material increases the differences in density between anatomic structures.
2. Intravenous iodine-based contrast carries the risks of causing acute renal failure and allergic reactions.

Head and Neck Imaging

TRAUMA

▓ FACIAL BONE FRACTURES

Anatomy

The facial bones and paranasal sinuses provide a natural "shock absorber," which, in addition to the calvaria, protects the brain during head trauma. The most commonly fractured skull bones are the nasal bones, maxillary antrum, walls of the orbit, and zygomatic arch (Figure 2-1).

Etiology

The two major categories of facial trauma are **blunt** and **penetrating** injuries. The most common causes of blunt trauma are motor-vehicle accidents (MVAs), falls, and assaults. Gunshot wounds are the most common penetrating traumas.

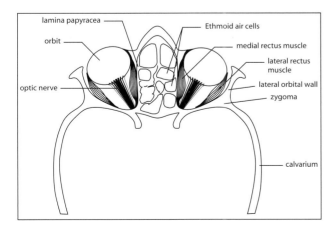

Figure 2-1 • Anatomy of facial bones at the level of the orbits.

Epidemiology

MVAs are the most common cause of facial trauma in young adults. In older adults, ground-level falls are the most common cause because they are unable to extend their arms to break the fall. Often patients in the hospital try to get out of bed in the middle of the night, become disoriented in the unfamiliar setting of their hospital room, and subsequently fall. Syncope, orthostatic hypotension, and weakness from prolonged bed rest place these patients at increased risk for a fall.

Clinical Manifestations

History

In MVAs, occult injuries occur more frequently in unrestrained passengers; so it is important to determine whether a patient was restrained or unrestrained. If the trauma occurred more than 24 hours before presentation, questions regarding headaches, visual changes, and sinus drainage become important because these symptoms may represent stable but significant facial trauma. Sinus drainage may be an indication of cerebrospinal fluid leakage from an open frontal or sphenoid sinus fracture. Open sinus fractures are extremely important to detect because they can lead to secondary intracerebral infections such as meningitis or abscess.

Physical Examination

Ecchymoses, soft-tissue swelling, and hematomas are the most common physical findings in facial trauma. Decreased visual acuity or strabismus are often present with orbital fractures and associated intraocular muscle or cranial nerve injury.

Diagnostic Evaluation

In acute trauma, the overall evaluation begins with an assessment of the patient's stability. Once airway, breathing, and circulation are established and a focused physical examination has been performed, the radiographic evaluation can begin. This evaluation, on rare occasions, when the case is uncomplicated, will begin with plain films; however, a noncontrast CT scan of the head is usually done to exclude intracranial injury in addition to facial fractures in a single examination. A head CT is especially important in patients with neurologic changes or decreased score on the Glasgow Coma Score (GCS) or Mini-Mental Status Examination (MMSE). Alterations in mental status may indicate intracranial injury that CT will detect, but plain films will not.

Radiologic Findings

The important areas on plain films are the orbits and the maxillary sinuses. "Blowout fractures" of the orbital floor are noted as a discontinuity of the bone cortex projecting into the ipsilateral maxillary sinus, best seen on a Caldwell-view plain film or a coronal view CT scan. An air-fluid level in the maxillary sinus, an associated finding in some cases, represents blood within the sinus. A soft-tissue mass projecting from the orbit into the maxillary sinus suggests herniation of the orbital soft tissues, and it is important to assess for entrapment of external ocular muscles.

Essential areas to evaluate on the head CT are the calvaria, orbital walls, paranasal sinuses, and mastoid air cells. Inspection of the calvaria includes bone and soft-tissue windows to look for fractures, soft-tissue swelling, and hematomas that would indicate areas of direct trauma. Subtle fractures are commonly found in the bone adjacent to areas of soft-tissue swelling. Assessment of the orbits by CT includes axial and coronal views with bone and soft-tissue windows. Coronal views are important to exclude orbital floor fractures, and soft-tissue windowing is crucial to exclude muscle entrapment or optic nerve impingement (Figures 2-2 and 2-3). In the paranasal sinuses, air-fluid levels of high attenuation represent acute blood (Figure 2-4), which is likely associated with subtle fractures. Fluid in the mastoid air cells is always pathologic; in the setting of trauma, it likely represents blood with an associated skull-base fracture (Figure 2-5).

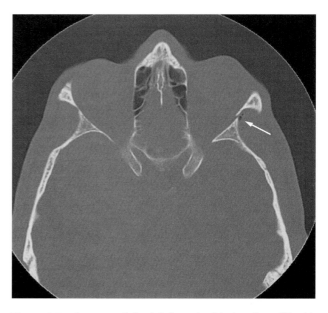

Figure 2-2 • Fracture of the left lateral orbital wall on CT with bone windows.
(Courtesy of Cedars-Sinai Medical Center, Los Angeles, CA.)

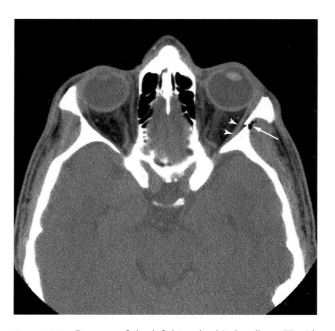

Figure 2-3 • Fracture of the left lateral orbital wall on CT with soft-tissue windows. There is close approximation of the fracture fragments to the lateral rectus muscle. In this case, there was no muscle entrapment.
(Courtesy of Cedars-Sinai Medical Center, Los Angeles, CA.)

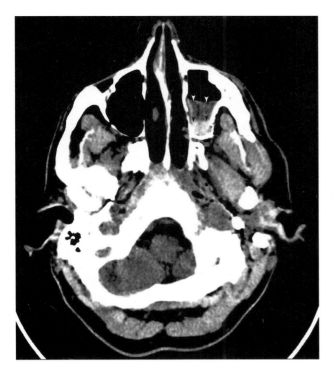

Figure 2-4 • CT of the head at the level of the maxillary sinuses reveals an air-fluid level in the left maxillary sinus. The fluid has two different densities, with higher density fluid layering dependently. This represents blood separated into plasma on top and red cells on the bottom.
(Courtesy of Cedars-Sinai Medical Center, Los Angeles, CA.)

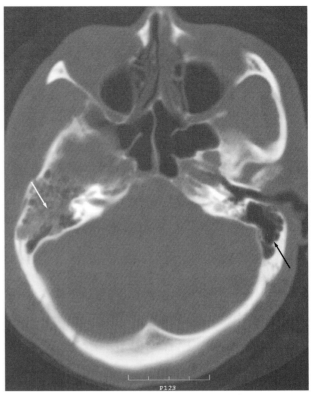

Figure 2-5 • CT of the head at the level of the skull base with bone windowing, demonstrating fluid in the patient's right mastoid air cells *(white arrow)* compared with the normal left side *(black arrow)*. The patient had an occult skull-base fracture.
(Courtesy of Cedars-Sinai Medical Center, Los Angeles, CA.)

KEY POINTS

1. Plain radiographs were previously the first step in the radiographic evaluation of facial trauma; however, a noncontrast CT scan of the head may preferentially be done to exclude facial fractures and intracranial injury in a single examination, especially in patients with changes in their mental status.
2. Air-fluid levels in the sinuses in the setting of trauma likely represent blood and indicate an occult fracture.
3. With orbital fractures, CT with bone and soft-tissue windows should be used to exclude muscle entrapment or optic nerve impingement.

◼ ACOUSTIC SCHWANNOMA/ VESTIBULOCOCHLEAR SCHWANNOMA

Anatomy

Cranial nerves VII and VIII run in the internal auditory canal (IAC), which angles horizontally from the cerebellopontine angle toward the petrous bone of the skull base. The open canal can usually be seen on at least one slice of a standard axial head CT (Figure 2-6). MRI is needed for fine detail of the nerves themselves (Figure 2-7).

Etiology

Acoustic schwannomas, also known as vestibulo-cochlear schwannomas or acoustic neuromas, arise from the Schwann cells of the axonal myelin sheaths. Schwannomas make up about 8% of all intracranial neoplasms and fall under the more general group of nerve sheath tumors, which also includes neurofibromas and malignant nerve sheath tumors.

Epidemiology

Most acoustic schwannomas occur de novo; however, neurofibromatosis (NF) is the condition most

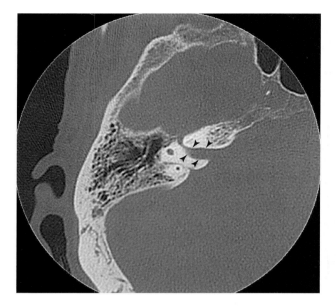

Figure 2-6 • CT of the head showing a normal right internal auditory canal.
(Courtesy of Cedars-Sinai Medical Center, Los Angeles, CA.)

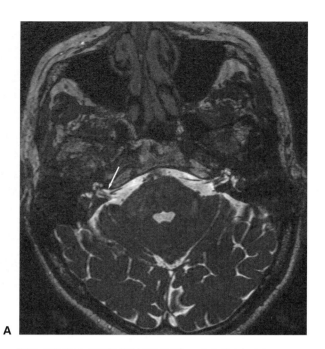

A

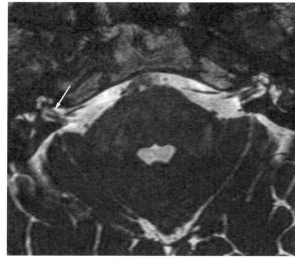

B

Figure 2-7 • **A:** MRI of the head with T2-weighting (cerebrospinal fluid is bright) showing normal course of cranial nerves VII and VIII into the internal auditory canals. **B:** Magnification view of (A).
(Courtesy of Cedars-Sinai Medical Center, Los Angeles, CA.)

commonly associated with them. NF type I (NF-I) represents 95% of the cases of neurofibromatosis and has an incidence of 1 in 2500 births. NF type II (NF-II) has an incidence of 1 in 50,000 and represents 5% of NF cases. However, if bilateral vestibular schwannomas are present, this is essentially pathognomonic for NF-II.

Clinical Manifestations

History

Patients complain of gradual-onset hearing loss, which may be unilateral or bilateral. Depending on the extent of the schwannoma, vertigo, tinnitus, or an internal ear infection may be present.

Physical Examination

Visual inspection of the external ear canal and tympanic membrane should be performed. Hearing and vibratory sensation can be tested with the Rinne and Weber tests using tuning forks of different frequencies. The eyes should be tested for nystagmus and, using an ophthalmoscope, for papilledema from hydrocephalus caused by obstruction of the normal flow of cerebrospinal fluid.

Diagnostic Evaluation

Contrast-enhanced CT scan of the head is an appropriate screening examination for suspected acoustic schwannoma. Osseous erosion is important for detect-

ing acoustic schwannoma on CT. MRI with gadolinium contrast is the imaging modality of choice. Thin sections (3 mm) through the temporal bone on CT or basal cisterns on MRI may be required for diagnosis.

Radiologic Findings

A brightly enhancing mass in the IAC or within the cerebellopontine angle is the most common finding of

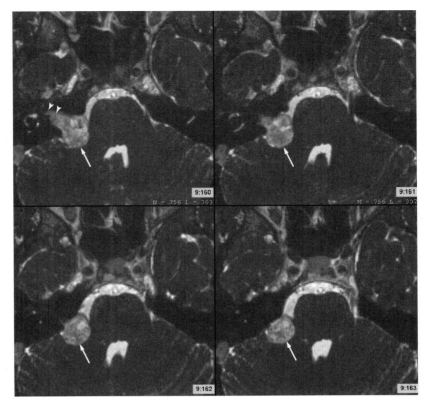

Figure 2-8 • Acoustic schwannoma *(arrows)* in the right cerebellopontine angle on T2-weighted MRI.
(Courtesy of Cedars-Sinai Medical Center, Los Angeles, CA.)

acoustic schwannoma and may be seen on either CT or MRI. A vestibular schwannoma may be difficult to distinguish from a meningioma, which classically has a broad dural tail that the schwannoma does not have. A meningioma forms a broad base with the adjacent bone, whereas the schwannoma does not. Acoustic schwannoma extends along the course of the seventh and eighth nerves, often into the IAC (Figure 2-8). The IAC will likely be enlarged because of gradual expansion of the tumor (Figure 2-9), which is best seen on CT with bone windowing. NF-I often has associated findings of optic gliomas, cerebral astrocytomas, scoliosis, and intraspinal neurofibromas. NF-II commonly has associated findings of multiple meningiomas and spinal nerve schwannomas.

▓ HEAD AND NECK CANCER

Anatomy

Mass lesions of the head and neck may be difficult to classify based on radiologic appearance alone,

KEY POINTS

1. Acoustic neuroma, more properly called a **vestibular schwannoma,** arises from Schwann cells, which constitute the myelin sheaths of axons.
2. Nearly all patients with bilateral acoustic schwannomas have NF-II.
3. Patients with acoustic schwannomas complain of gradual-onset hearing loss.
4. An enhancing mass in the internal auditory canal or within the cerebellopontine angle on either CT or MRI is the most common finding of vestibular schwannoma.
5. MRI is the imaging modality of choice.

but the differential diagnosis can be narrowed by identifying the adjacent anatomic structures and determining the most likely tissue type of origin. The most common sites of head and neck cancer are the vocal cords, the pterygopalatine fossa, the

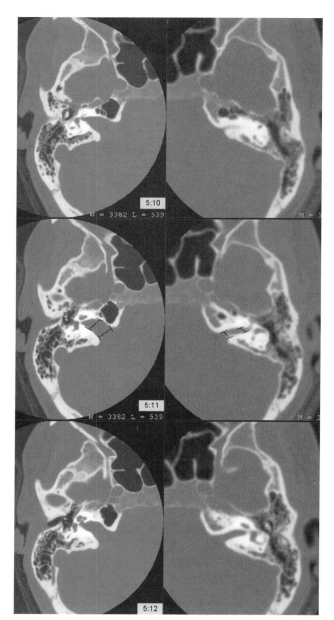

Figure 2-9 • Expansion of right internal auditory canal by acoustic schwannoma on CT with bone windowing.
(Courtesy of Cedars-Sinai Medical Center, Los Angeles, CA.)

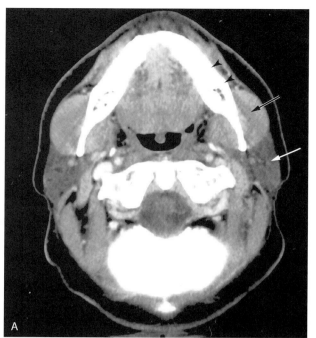

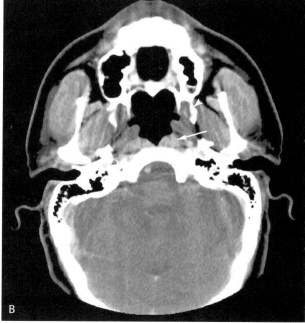

Figure 2-10 • A: Normal CT scan of the head with soft-tissue windowing at the level of the parotid glands *(white arrow).* (Mandibular ramus, *arrowheads;* masseter muscle, *black arrows.*) **B:** Normal CT of the head at the level of the pterygoid plates *(arrowhead)* and nasopharyngeal soft tissues *(white arrow).*
(Courtesy of Cedars-Sinai Medical Center, Los Angeles, CA.)

cavernous sinus, and the nasopharyngeal soft tissues (Figure 2-10).

Etiology

Three basic tissue types give rise to most head and neck malignancies: squamous epithelium, lymphoid tissue, and salivary glands. Squamous cell carcinoma is by far the most common type of head and neck cancer. The salivary glands may also have tumors that are specific to each gland. For example, the parotid gland commonly has benign tumors (80%), such as pleomorphic adenomas and Warthin tumors. The parotid gland also has malignant tumors (20%), such as adenocarcinoma, adenocystic carcinoma, squamous cell carcinoma, and mucoepidermoid carcinoma. Thyroid neoplasms may be benign (e.g., thyroid adenoma) or malignant (e.g., follicular, papillary, anaplastic carcinoma).

Epidemiology

Head and neck cancers generally occur in the fourth to eighth decades. These cancers occur more commonly in men.

Pathogenesis

The occurrence of head and neck cancers is attributed to smoking, drinking, and oral tobacco use. There is also an increased risk of thyroid cancer with prior radiation exposure.

Clinical Manifestations

History

Symptoms depend on the location, origin, and type of tumor. Patients with squamous cell carcinoma of the pharynx complain of nasal obstruction, epistaxis, facial pain, or headache. Tumors of the larynx often cause hoarseness, changes in voice tone, or dysphagia. Lymphoma frequently presents with constitutional symptoms such as fever, fatigue, and weight loss in addition to cervical lymph node enlargement.

Physical Examination

Examination of the throat commonly reveals a mass arising from the palate or within the nasopharynx. Palpation of enlarged cervical lymph nodes is frequent.

Radiologic Findings

Both CT and MRI can be used to examine the head and neck. MRI has the advantage of excellent soft-tissue contrast and demonstration of the extent of a soft-tissue mass. CT has the advantage of detecting

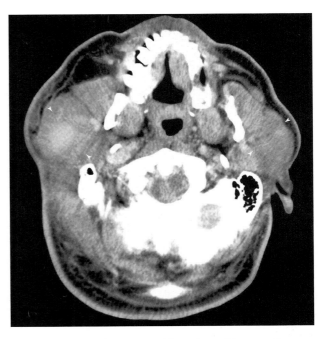

Figure 2-11 • Parotid carcinoma. Bilateral parotid masses *(between arrowheads)* seen on contrast-enhanced CT scan of the neck. There are areas of necrosis suggesting rapid growth of the tumor, which has outgrown its blood supply.
(Courtesy of Cedars-Sinai Medical Center, Los Angeles, CA.)

involvement of osseous structures with osseous erosion or abnormalities of the paranasal sinuses.

Disruption of normal anatomic spaces and vascular relationships is a useful finding when surveying the extent of a tumor and may give clues as to its origin. For example, a tumor of the parotid gland may push the carotid artery posteriorly or medially (Figure 2-11). A tumor of the pterygopalatine fossa may be seen on physical examination or on CT of the head to expand the soft palate inferiorly or medially (Figure 2-12). Malignant neoplasms generally invade

KEY POINTS

1. Squamous cell carcinoma is the most common type of head and neck cancer.
2. Contrast-enhanced CT and MRI each have advantages for assessment of head and neck cancer.
3. Disruption of normal anatomic spaces and vascular relationships is a useful finding when surveying the extent and origin of a tumor.

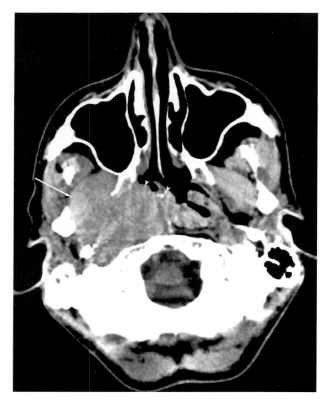

Figure 2-12 • Pterygopalatine fossa carcinoma. CT scan of the neck demonstrates a large right pterygopalatine fossa mass. (Arrow and arrowheads delineate the medial and lateral extent of tumor.)
(Courtesy of Cedars-Sinai Medical Center, Los Angeles, CA.)

bone, and interrupted bone cortices may be seen on bone windows. Benign masses may remodel bone but leave the cortices intact.

■ RETROPHARYNGEAL ABSCESS

Anatomy

The retropharyngeal space (RPS) is located midline between the airway and the prevertebral fascia, and it extends from the base of the skull to the upper mediastinum. The lymph nodes in the retropharyngeal space drain the posterior nasal passage, nasopharynx, middle ear, and palatine tonsils. The danger is spread through the retropharyngeal space into the mediastinum, causing mediastinitis, and through the "danger space" (a subspace that extends to the diaphragm). Mediastinitis is not only a surgical emergency, but it is also a high-mortality complication. The other complication is internal jugular vein thrombosis

resulting from the anatomic proximity of the retropharyngeal space to the vascular structures (carotid space).

Etiology

Retropharyngeal abscesses commonly follow a bacterial pharyngitis, upper respiratory tract infection, or dental abscess. Group A *Streptococcus (Streptococcus pyogenes)* is usually responsible for peritonsillar and retropharyngeal abscesses. Tuberculosis is also reported in adults. Figure 2-13 shows a left peritonsillar abscess extending into the retropharyngeal space.

Epidemiology

Retropharyngeal abscesses occur most commonly in children and are uncommon in adults (other than post penetrating trauma or dental abscesses).

Pathogenesis

Infection spreads from the upper airway via lymphatics. Because the lymphoid tissue is more prominent in

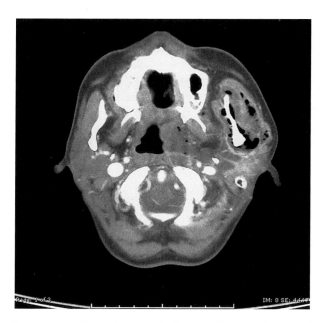

Figure 2-13 • Retropharyngeal abscess. CT scan of the neck demonstrates a left peritonsillar abscess containing gas and extending into the left masticator space and retropharyngeal space to the superior mediastinum.
(Courtesy of University of Southern California Medical Center, Los Angeles, CA.)

children (i.e., adenoids), they are more prone to retropharyngeal abscesses. Pus from the space posterior to the prevertebral fascia perforates into the retropharyngeal space.

Clinical Manifestations

History

Neck stiffness, fever, odynophagia, and dysphagia are common symptoms associated with retropharyngeal abscess.

Physical Examination

On physical examination, posterior pharyngeal erythema and edematous mucosa are observed. Children may drool.

Diagnostic Evaluation

Retropharyngeal abscess can be detected on plain radiographs on lateral view of soft tissues of the neck. CT with contrast delineates the anatomy and demonstrates the extent of abscess.

Radiologic Findings

If lucencies are seen on plain radiographs within the enlarged prevertebral soft tissues, gas is present within the abscess. Caution should be exercised in assessing the prevertebral soft-tissue thickness in flexion in children (flexion of the cervical spine may lead to erroneous diagnosis by resulting in an apparent retropharyngeal mass). Usually the retropharyngeal abscess results in loss of the normal cervical spine lordosis as a result of patient discomfort.

Using CT, administration of contrast also can distinguish cellulitis from abscess by demonstrating ring enhancement, and this makes a fluid collection more conspicuous.

Differential Diagnosis

Once gas is present in the lesion, an abscess should be diagnosed. Other diagnoses should be considered if no gas is identified (e.g., hemangioma, lymphangioma, other neoplasms).

Treatment

Surgical incision and drainage are the standard treatment, but caution should be exercised (contrast-enhanced CT of the neck is recommended to determine the course of the carotid arteries because of their proximity to the retropharyngeal space).

KEY POINTS

1. Retropharyngeal abscess is a serious condition, as its complications can be lethal (mediastinitis).
2. On lateral neck plain radiograph small lucencies represent gas bubbles within an abscess.
3. A CT with intravenous contrast is recommended to determine the extent of disease and to delineate the anatomy for incision and drainage.

■ SINUSITIS

Inflammation of the paranasal sinuses occurs secondary to bacterial, viral, and fungal infections or allergies.

Anatomy

The paranasal sinuses are extensions of the nasal cavity into the maxillary, ethmoid, sphenoid, and frontal bones, and they derive from ectoderm. Pneumatization of the paranasal sinuses begins at different times, occurs slowly in childhood, and progresses to completion at different ages (maxillary sinuses become entirely pneumatized by 12 years of age, the ethmoid air cells by 18 years of age, frontal and sphenoid sinuses by adulthood). Usually the mucus secreted by the mucosal glands of the paranasal sinuses drains into the superior or lateral nose through the ostia.

Etiology

In adults, the most common organisms are *Streptococcus pneumoniae* and *Haemophilus influenzae*. In children, *Moraxella catarrhalis* should also be considered in choosing therapy. Chronic sinusitis commonly yields gram-negative rods or anaerobic organisms. Acute sinusitis is bacterial (or fungal in immunocompromised patients).

Fungal sinusitis has high mortality and is categorized as **noninvasive** (in immunocompetent hosts) or **invasive** (in immunodeficient and immunocompetent patients). Fungi often proliferate after an insufficiently treated bacterial sinusitis; the most common are *Aspergillus*, *Candida*, and the *Mucor* organisms.

Epidemiology

Sinusitis occurs in both immunocompetent and immunocompromised patients. Fungal infections are common in immunocompromised patients.

Pathogenesis

Viral infections inflame the nasal mucosa and obstruct the sinus ostia, resulting in superimposed bacterial infections. Infection of the paranasal sinuses also occurs from extension of infection from the nasal passage through the meatus of each sinus. The maxillary sinus infections may also occur as a result of extension of maxillary teeth.

Clinical Manifestations

History

Sinusitis manifests with nasal congestion and local pain (worsens when the patient bends over or lies supine). Fever develops in about 50% of patients with acute sinusitis. Infection of the ethmoid air cells may break through the thin medial orbital wall (lamina papyracea) and extend into the orbit (resulting in cellulitis or abscess) and into the optic canal, sometimes causing even blindness. Occurrence of osteomyelitis is not infrequent.

Of even greater concern is intracranial extension of infection resulting in epidural abscess, subdural empyema (pus between the dura and arachnoid causes seizures, headache, lethargy), meningitis (meningeal signs, e.g., neck stiffness), intracerebral abscess (lethargy, seizures), and cavernous sinus thrombophlebitis (proptosis, papilledema, cranial nerve palsies III, IV, V, and VI).

Physical Examination

The invasive fungal sinusitis has an indolent course in immunocompetent patients, whereas in immunocompromised patients, it has an acute presentation. Black eschars within the nasal passages are found within mucormycosis, and extensive surgical debridement is needed as the fungus erodes adjacent bone and spreads rapidly.

Diagnostic Evaluation

Plain radiographs are no longer considered the standard of care because CT provides the appropriate axial and coronal planes' details. CT is used in cases that are complicated, severe, long standing, or unresponsive to medical therapy. Imaging is needed to ensure an absence of granulomatous disease (e.g., tuberculosis) and tumor obstructing the drainage of sinuses. Noncontrast-enhanced CT is commonly performed, but if tumor is suspected based on images, contrast should be administered.

Radiologic Findings

Air-fluid levels and gas bubbles are seen in acute sinusitis. Fluid levels, mucosal thickening, and opacification of sinuses are diagnostic. However, it is thought that many patients have mucosal thickening from a common cold or allergies without having sinusitis.

Fungal sinusitis demonstrates higher than soft-tissue attenuation (i.e., has areas of increased density or white within the sinus fluid collection) (Figure 2-14). In invasive fungal sinusitis, frequent follow-up CT or MRI is recommended.

Expansion of the sinus walls with thinning of bone and complete filling of the cavity with mucus characterizes a mucocele, which is a result of long-standing sinus drainage obstruction (Figure 2-15).

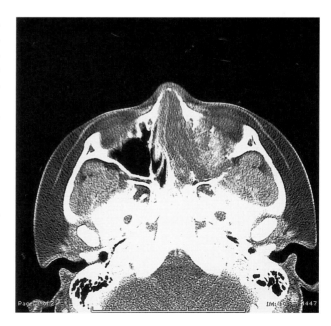

Figure 2-14 • Fungal sinusitis. High-attenuation material is present in the left maxillary sinus.
(Courtesy of University of Southern California Medical Center, Los Angeles, CA.)

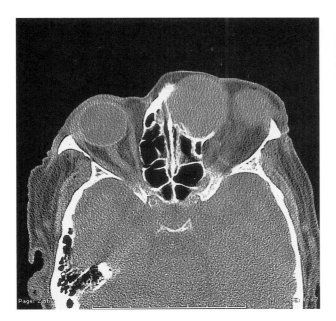

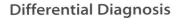

Figure 2-15 • Left ethmoid sinus mucocele. Noncontrast-enhanced CT scan shows that the left ethmoid air cells walls are expanded and contain inspissated mucus.
(Courtesy of University of Southern California Medical Center, Los Angeles, CA.)

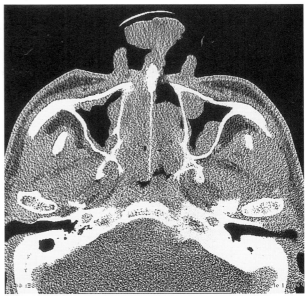

Figure 2-16 • Polypoid rhinosinusitis. Pansinus mucosal hypertrophy of the paranasal sinuses into hypervascular masses is present. Sinus polyposis is coexistent with infectious sinusitis and is considered as a result of long-standing inflammation (infection, allergic reactions, smoking, etc.). The maxillary sinuses and the nasal cavity contain the previously described masses. (Note the concurrent patient's nasal soft tissue superficial tumor, which was proven to be a squamous cell carcinoma.)
(Courtesy of University of Southern California Medical Center, Los Angeles, CA.)

Differential Diagnosis

Granulomatous disease, polypoid rhinosinusitis, benign and malignant tumors, and granulomatous diseases (e.g., tuberculosis [TB], syphilis, sarcoidosis) result in destructive changes of the sinus walls, simulating malignancy. Polypoid rhinosinusitis (polyposis) is characterized by mucosal thickening resulting in masses (**pseudopolyps**) (Figure 2-16). Benign tumors can be distinguished from malignant ones by having an indolent course and by being more likely to cause expansion of bone without erosion.

Treatment

Empiric medical treatment only is initiated in mild cases. Severe acute sinusitis may need endoscopic surgical intervention consisting of enlarging the ostia and facilitating drainage of the sinuses.

Noninvasive aspergilloma requires surgical treatment only. Invasive fungal sinusitis requires debridement and intravenous amphotericin B.

KEY POINTS

1. In complicated cases of sinusitis (i.e., prolonged or severe), CT of the sinuses is the standard of care for diagnostic imaging. Plain films, although they may demonstrate air-fluid levels in the sinuses in some cases of acute sinusitis, are no longer recommended.
2. Intravenous contrast is not routinely used for CT. Its use is limited to patients with suspected tumor or for preoperative planning in severe cases of sinusitis.
3. Air-fluid levels in sinuses diagnose acute sinusitis.
4. Mucosal thickening is seen not only in chronic sinusitis but also with allergies or mild viral infections.

Neurologic Imaging

ANATOMY AND GENERAL PRINCIPLES

The differential diagnosis for intracranial and intraspinal lesions, like that of head and neck pathology, is determined by both anatomic location and imaging characteristics. A neoplasm in the posterior fossa entails a different diagnostic approach than one in the middle cranial fossa or suprasellar region. Anatomically, intracranial pathology is defined as either intra-axial or extra-axial, which is the first step in narrowing the differential diagnosis. The term **intra-axial** refers to any lesion within the brain parenchyma. **Extra-axial** refers to a lesion outside the brain parenchyma itself and may be between any layer of the meninges. Along the same line of reasoning, lesions within the spinal canal are classified as **intramedullary** or **extramedullary, intradural** or **extradural.** Important imaging characteristics in neuroradiology include lesion size, shape, attenuation on CT, and signal characteristics on MRI. Contrast enhancement is an important characteristic for both modalities.

CT and MRI constitute most neuroradiologic examinations. Plain films are rarely used except for suspected skull fractures and occasional screening studies of the paranasal sinuses. CT is an effective screening examination for intracranial pathology, especially in trauma and emergent situations, because it has a high sensitivity for detecting acute bleeding and fractures, and it can be performed and interpreted rapidly. A CT examination can be completed within a few minutes, whereas an MRI may require anywhere from 30 minutes to several hours to complete.

MRI is superior to CT in many situations, including evaluation of the posterior fossa, the detection of subtle lesions not associated with hemorrhage or significant edema, and detection of spinal cord lesions. MRA is also a useful, noninvasive technique to survey the intracranial vasculature for vascular malformations and aneurysms. MRI and MRA are often used for follow-up examinations when a head CT is abnormal. Images are acquired in multiple planes (axial, sagittal, and coronal), unlike CT, which is generally limited to the transverse plane. MRI is commonly obtained as the initial test for suspected brain neoplasm and as a follow-up examination for known pathology, such as a suspected tumor recurrence or prior stroke.

KEY POINTS

1. The differential diagnosis for intracranial and intraspinal lesions is determined by both anatomic location and imaging characteristics.
2. **Intra-axial** refers to any lesion within the brain or spinal cord parenchyma, and **extra-axial** refers to any lesion outside the brain parenchyma.
3. CT is ideal for emergency situations because it has a high sensitivity and can be performed and interpreted rapidly.
4. MRI generally has a higher specificity for intracranial abnormalities because it can detect subtle pathology in the brain and cerebral vasculature.
5. MRI produces images in multiple planes (axial, sagittal, and coronal).

HEAD TRAUMA

EPIDURAL HEMATOMA

Anatomy

An **epidural hematoma** is defined as an extra-axial hemorrhage within the potential space between the inner table of the calvaria and the outer layer of the dura mater. The outer layer of the dura is fused to the calvaria at the suture margins, which makes it impossible for an epidural hematoma to cross them.

Etiology

The cause is most often blunt trauma and injury to the middle meningeal artery (90% of cases).

Epidemiology

Epidural hematoma occurs in about 2% of all head injuries.

Clinical Manifestations

History

The history may be any type of head trauma but commonly involves an MVA in young patients or a ground-level fall in older patients. A key point in the history is a "lucid interval," in which the patient has a near-normal MMSE early after a trauma but subsequently has delayed-onset decreased level of consciousness. This alteration of consciousness corresponds to progression and enlargement of the epidural hematoma with associated compression of adjacent brain structures.

Physical Examination

Focal neurologic deficits and unequal pupils are commonly found, depending on the severity of the injury. Systemic hypertension is an uncommon but serious associated finding with increased intracranial pressure.

Diagnostic Evaluation

If an epidural hematoma is suspected, an emergent CT scan without contrast is necessary. Once an epidural hematoma is diagnosed, serial CT scans are usually performed for monitoring, with or without neurosurgical intervention.

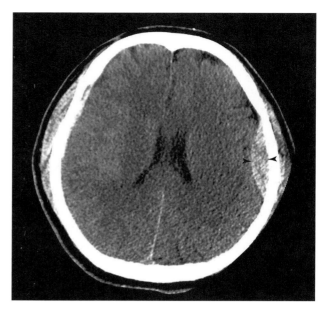

Figure 3-1 • Epidural hematoma. Classic findings on CT scan of lens-shaped, high-attenuation collection in left frontal region. (Courtesy of Cedars-Sinai Medical Center, Los Angeles, CA.)

Radiologic Findings

Acute blood appears as a **high attenuation,** or bright area, on CT. An epidural hematoma has a classic biconvex (lens-shaped) appearance (Figure 3-1) that does not cross suture lines, as subdural hematomas sometimes do. An epidural hematoma occasionally crosses the midline falx cerebri, however, whereas subdural hematomas never do. Mass effect on the adjacent brain parenchyma, often with compression of the lateral ventricles, is frequently seen with large epidural hematomas, and 95% of patients with an epidural hematoma have an associated adjacent skull fracture.

KEY POINTS

1. An **epidural hematoma** is an extra-axial hemorrhage within the potential space between the inner table of the calvaria and the outer layer of the dura mater.
2. Epidural hematomas do not cross suture lines, but they may cross the midline.
3. The classic appearance of an epidural hematoma on a noncontrast CT of the brain is a high-attenuation, lens-shaped focal collection of blood.

■ SUBDURAL HEMATOMA

Anatomy

A **subdural hematoma** is a collection of blood within the potential space between the dura mater and the pia mater.

Etiology

Common causes of subdural hematoma are acute deceleration injuries, such as an MVE or fall. They are often seen in patients who are on anticoagulation for other medical conditions. Patients taking warfarin or heparin are at highest risk. Aspirin, taken daily by patients with coronary artery disease, slightly increases the risk of developing a subdural hematoma after even minor trauma.

Epidemiology

Subdural hematomas occur in 5% of all traumatic head injuries. They are often seen in older patients after a fall or in children following blunt trauma. In children, subdural hematomas are the most common intracranial complication from child abuse ("shaken baby syndrome").

Pathogenesis

Acute subdural hematomas are the result of damage to bridging veins that cross from the brain cortex to the venous sinuses. Chronic subdural hematomas result from a repeating cycle of recurrent bleeding into the subdural space and resorption of the resultant hematoma.

Clinical Manifestations

History

Of patients with symptomatic subdural hematomas, 99% have an altered level of consciousness within minutes to hours after the causative injury.

Physical Examination

Presenting signs are hemiparesis, unilateral pupillary dilatation, and papilledema.

Diagnostic Evaluation

A noncontrast CT scan of the head is the imaging modality of choice for acute and chronic subdural hematomas.

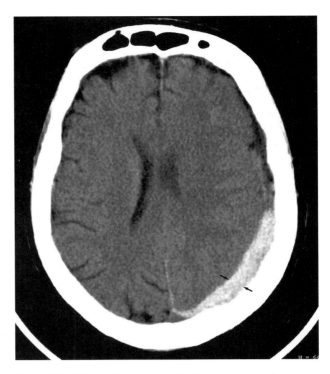

Figure 3-2 • Subdural hematoma. Classic appearance of crescent-shaped subdural hematoma on CT with high-attenuation collection in left frontoparietal region, which crosses the lambdoid suture.
(Courtesy of Cedars-Sinai Medical Center, Los Angeles, CA.)

Radiologic Findings

The classic CT finding is a crescent-shaped area of high attenuation that may cross suture lines (Figure 3-2). Subacute (>1 week) and early chronic (>3 to 4 weeks) hematomas may have a fluid-fluid level where the lower attenuation serum is separated from the higher attenuation cellular portion of blood. If the patient's hemoglobin level is less than 9, blood appears isointense or even hypointense to adjacent brain and a hematoma will be difficult to distinguish. In this case, iodine contrast may be given to increase the contrast between the hematoma and subjacent brain tissue.

■ INTRACEREBRAL HEMATOMA

Anatomy

Intracerebral hematomas occur within the brain parenchyma and gray or white matter.

Etiology and Pathogenesis

Intracerebral hematomas occur mostly following trauma but may be seen with other conditions, such as vascular malformations, tumors, hypertension, and amyloidosis. In cases following trauma, coup- and contrecoup-type injuries are classically seen. The **coup injury** is due to acute deceleration and shearing of small intracerebral blood vessels. The **contrecoup injury** is the secondary brain injury seen at the portion of the brain opposite the vector of impact and is specifically referred to as a **cortical contusion** because it affects the superficial gray matter. A contrecoup injury occurs when the rebound force from the direct injury propels the brain in the opposite direction, causing it to impact against the inner table of the skull.

Other nontraumatic causes of intraparenchymal hemorrhage may occur in any portion of the brain but often have an anatomic predilection, depending on the underlying cause. Hemorrhage resulting from hypertension classically occurs in the basal ganglia. Vascular malformations (Figure 3-3) are typically supratentorial but may occur in any location. Intraparenchymal hemorrhage resulting in amyloidosis typically occurs in the occipital and parietal lobes. Bleeding from a primary brain tumor or metastatic lesion may occur within or around the tumor. Metastatic renal cell carcinoma (Figure 3-4) and melanoma are two tumors that have a high predilection for bleeding.

Clinical Manifestations

History

Patients with an intracerebral hematoma from trauma often have sudden loss of consciousness immediately following the traumatic event. Nontraumatic causes of intraparenchymal hemorrhage frequently present with focal neurologic signs, loss of consciousness, and labored breathing.

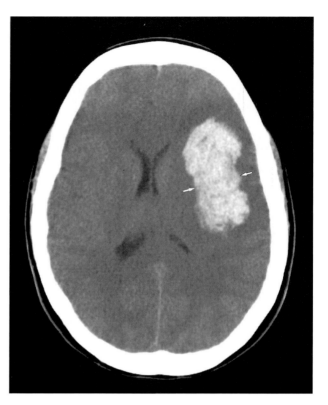

Figure 3-3 • Intracerebral hematoma. This noncontrast CT image demonstrates blood within the left frontal lobe, which originated from an arteriovenous malformation. The patient presented with confusion and right hemiplegia.
(Courtesy of Cedars-Sinai Medical Center, Los Angeles, CA.)

Physical Examination

Pupillary dilatation (often unilateral) and changes in GCS are the most common physical findings. The GCS takes into account eye opening, motor response, and verbal response.

Diagnostic Evaluation

Noncontrast CT of the brain should be ordered for emergent diagnosis of extent of hemorrhage. Repeated CT examinations are performed for assessment of bleeding extent and progression.

Radiologic Findings

Findings associated with an intracerebral hematoma depend primarily on the cause. Trauma-induced hematomas commonly are multiple small, well-demarcated areas of high attenuation within brain

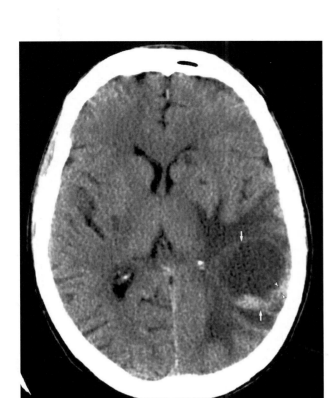

Figure 3-4 • Metastatic lesion with hemorrhage. Noncontrast CT scan of the brain demonstrates a 4-cm left posterior parietal cystic mass *(arrows)* with areas of hemorrhage *(arrowheads)* and surrounding cytotoxic edema. This patient had a history of renal cell carcinoma, and the lesion was a metastasis.
(Courtesy of Cedars-Sinai Medical Center, Los Angeles, CA.)

parenchyma on CT. These are often surrounded by a rim of hypoattenuation, representing edema from adjacent damaged cells. Mass effect is common and is seen as compression of the ventricular system and shift of the third ventricle and falx to the contralateral side. Secondary localized edema with midline shift places the patient at increased risk for subtentorial or subfalcine brain herniation and subsequent brain death.

KEY POINTS

1. Intracerebral hematomas occur mostly following trauma, but they may be seen with other conditions, such as vascular malformations, tumors, hypertension, and amyloidosis.
2. Trauma-induced hematomas commonly are multiple small, well-demarcated areas of high attenuation within brain parenchyma on CT.

STROKE

Anatomy

The three major paired arteries that supply the brain are the anterior, middle, and posterior cerebral arteries (ACA, MCA, and PCA). The ACA and MCA arteries are branches of the internal carotid arteries, and the paired PCAs are the terminal branches of the vertebrobasilar arterial tree.

Etiology

Patients with atrial fibrillation and atherosclerotic disease are at high risk for thromboemboli to occlude one of the main intracranial arteries. Aortic dissection that extends into the carotid arteries is also a cause of stroke.

Epidemiology

In older adults, stroke is the second leading cause of morbidity and mortality, behind only ischemic cardiac disease.

Pathogenesis

Events of MCA are the most common and the most devastating. Occasionally the associated edema results in cerebellar tonsil or uncal herniation, brainstem compression, and death. Often patients survive but are left with a hemiparesis or other serious neurologic deficit.

Clinical Manifestations

History

Complaints of unilateral weakness, numbness, or tingling are the most common presentations of stroke. If the diagnosis of nonhemorrhagic cerebral ischemia or infarct can be made, then a stroke treatment protocol can be initiated early to minimize the permanent damage.

Physical Examination

The neurologic examination often demonstrates contralateral weakness or flaccid paralysis, facial droop, slurred speech, and ptosis.

Diagnostic Evaluation

CT without contrast is the most rapid imaging study in suspected cases of stroke. MRI with diffusion-weighted imaging (DWI) is a highly sensitive and specific test for cerebral infarction in the first 6 hours. Because MRI is becoming more accessible and the time of examination shorter, it is predicted that it will replace CT for early detection of ischemic events.

Radiologic Findings

Early in a stroke, the noncontrast CT of the brain will likely appear normal. It is important to exclude associated intracerebral hemorrhage, which would preclude antithrombotic treatment. Within a few hours, subtle findings emerge, including loss of a distinct gray-white junction and blurring of the cortical sulci in the affected vascular distribution. Following thromboembolic strokes, low-attenuation areas of edema within a vascular territory define the culprit vessel (Figure 3-5). Potential complications of stroke include delayed hemorrhage in the infarcted tissue, mass effect from the associated edema, and herniation with permanent brain damage or death. DWI reveals bright signal intensity in the affected territory of the stroke (Figure 3-6).

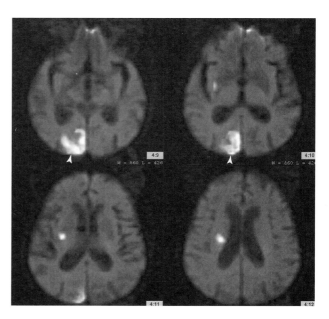

Figure 3-6 • Stroke. A MRI with DWI reveals an area of high signal intensity *(arrowheads)* in the right occipital lobe consistent with acute infarct in the right posterior cerebral artery distribution. (Courtesy of Cedars-Sinai Medical Center, Los Angeles, CA.)

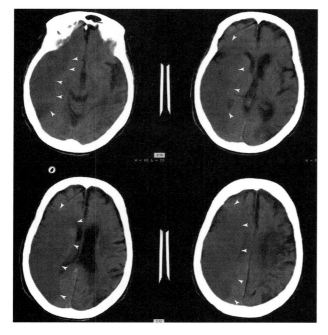

Figure 3-5 • Stroke. Noncontrast CT scan of the brain demonstrates a large area of hypoattenuation-dark (ischemia) *(arrowheads)* spanning the distribution of the MCA. A prior left MCA infarct with encephalomalacia is also present. (Courtesy of Cedars-Sinai Medical Center, Los Angeles, CA.)

KEY POINTS

1. Most cases of stroke are caused by thromboemboli.
2. Early in a stroke, the noncontrast CT of the brain will likely appear normal.
3. If a stroke is suspected, it is important to exclude an intracranial hemorrhage.
4. Loss of a distinct gray-white junction and blurring of the cortical sulci in the affected vascular distribution are subtle findings that appear within several hours.
5. MRI with DWI is a highly sensitive and specific test for stroke.

■ BRAIN NEOPLASMS

Any growing brain mass can have a neoplastic, infectious, hemorrhagic etiology or represent a vascular malformation. Brain neoplasms are primary (70%) or metastatic (30%). As mentioned at the beginning of the chapter, it is important to distinguish between intra-axial and extra-axial neoplasms to narrow the differential diagnosis and for preoperative planning. The distinction, however, is not always attainable. A relatively short discussion is provided in this book to familiarize the reader with brain neoplasms.

Etiology

Some of the benign brain tumors have known association with syndromes (e.g., acoustic neuromas), but most brain neoplasms have unknown etiology.

Epidemiology

Adult versus child and some female versus male brain tumor differences exist. **Childhood tumors** are most commonly located in the posterior cranial fossa. Primary brain neoplasms in children are cerebellar astrocytoma and medulloblastoma, ependymomas (which arise from the ventricles or the central canal of spinal cord lining), gliomas (optic nerve and brainstem), germinomas, and congenital tumors. Metastases to the epidural space originate most commonly from neuroblastoma (malignant neoplasm arising from neuroblasts, 30% of which occur in the adrenal glands) and to the meninges from leukemia or lymphoma.

Adult common tumors include meningioma, schwannomas (see acoustic schwannoma discussion in Chapter 2), primary lymphomas (seen in acquired immunodeficiency disease syndrome [AIDS] patients and older adults), and gliomas. Meningiomas (which are believed to have progesterone receptors and grow during pregnancy) and schwannomas have a female preponderance; glioblastoma multiforme (high-grade, undifferentiated glioma) has predilection for males. Brain metastases originate from lung, breast, melanoma, etc.

Clinical Manifestations

History

Symptoms are various and range from headache, personality changes, and vomiting (morning vomiting is attributed to increased intracranial pressure during the night secondary to prolonged supine position) to seizures, lethargy, and even respiratory and cardiac arrest (from brainstem herniation due to mass effect).

Physical Examination

Focal neurologic deficits may alert a clinician to location of a lesion and to its existence. For example, pituitary macroadenomas present with loss of peripheral vision (bitemporal hemianopsia). Young children may present with large head circumference because of increased intracranial pressure (failure of suture closure).

Diagnostic Evaluation

Monitoring of brain neoplasms after surgical and medical intervention is routine. MRI with gadolinium is used, but many times tumor recurrence cannot be distinguished from postsurgical inflammatory changes. PET is gaining ground in making this distinction (neoplasms have high metabolism and demonstrate high uptake of radiotracer).

A CT of the chest, abdomen, and pelvis before surgical resection of a brain tumor is sometimes requested by neurosurgeons. If the brain lesion is a metastasis (i.e., from lymphoma), medical treatment should be instituted (chemotherapy) instead of an aggressive futile neurosurgical intervention.

Radiologic Findings

Gadolinium-enhanced MRI is the standard imaging modality with good anatomic delineation (Figures 3-7); iodinated contrast-enhanced CT may be a fast, easily accessible modality, but it is not definitive. The anatomic information limitations of CT and the risks of iodinated contrast administration (see Chapter 1) should make contrast CT use restricted to emergencies. The more aggressive the intracranial tumor, the more enhancement is present as a result of the disruption of blood-brain barrier (the newly formed blood vessels feeding the neoplasm lack the native brain vessels' properties).

MRI spectroscopy is becoming better understood and is used for differentiating not only between malignancy and benign tumors but also between recurrence of tumor versus radiation necrosis (posttreatment changes). MRI spectroscopy is based on the metabolites present. A graph is plotted for a small volume of brain (voxel), and peaks of different metabolites are displayed. A high choline peak (choline is present in the cell membrane) on a graph correlates to an aggressive tumor.

Hydrocephalus associated with brain neoplasms is due to obstruction or mass effect of tumor on the ventricles, foraminae, or sylvian acqueduct (Figures 3-8). PET CT is increasingly used to monitor for recurrence of tumor as the radioactive isotopes are taken up by metabolically active tumor cells. It is expected

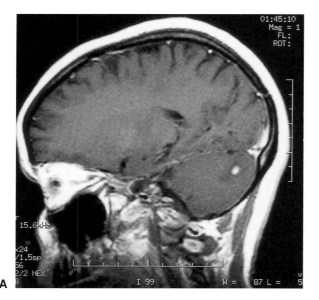
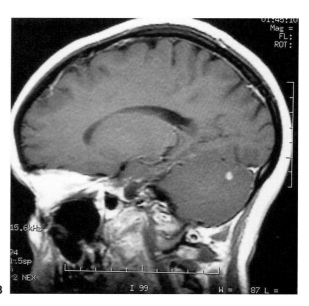

Figure 3-7 • Hemangioblastomas. (A & B) Sagittal T1-weighted MRI of the brain demonstrates small cerebellar-enhancing lesions (postgadolinium administration). This patient had a known history of von Hippel-Lindau syndrome. Hemangioblastomas need to be surgically excised in their entirety to prevent recurrence.
(Courtesy of University of Southern California Medical Center, Los Angeles, CA.)

that new MRI-enabling techniques will also be able to distinguish between recurrence in the tumor bed and postsurgical changes.

Primary brain neoplasms may be difficult to differentiate from one another. However, a few common tumor descriptions and typical locations are known.

Gliomas

Gliomas encompass the following tumors: astrocytomas, oligodendrogliomas, ependymomas, and medulloblastomas. An aggressive tumor of the cerebrum is glioblastoma multiforme (high-grade astrocytoma)

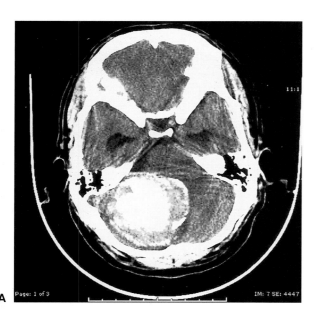
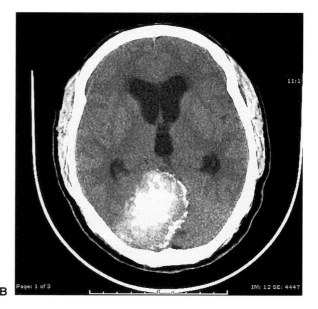

Figure 3-8 • Mass effect with resultant ventricular enlargement (lateral [A] and third ventricles [B]).
(Courtesy of University of Southern California Medical Center, Los Angeles, CA.)

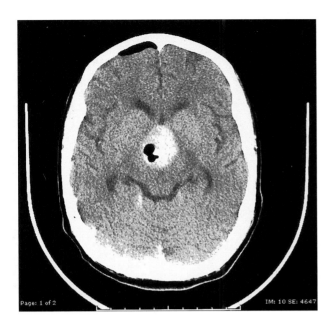

Figure 3-9 • Noncontrast CT scan of the brain demonstrates a third-ventricle tumor of high density (white) containing a dark area centrally (gas introduced into the tumor at stereotactic biopsy). Gas (pneumocephalus) is also present in the right anterior cranial fossa. A small volume of intracranial gas can be of no clinical consequence (e.g., when introduced by lumbar puncture). Final pathology diagnosed an astrocytoma.
(Courtesy of University of Southern California Medical Center, Los Angeles, CA.)

and presents as a large mass with central necrosis and peripheral edema (Figure 3-9). Ependymomas (originate from the ventricular lining) and oligodendrogliomas tend to calcify. Medulloblastomas arise from the roof of the IV ventricle. Primary brain lymphoma is located periventricularly.

Intraventricular Tumors

Besides ependymoma and medulloblastoma, intraventricular meningioma (a slow growing tumor arising from meninges) and hemangioblastoma are seen. In children, choroid plexus papilloma and its malignant corresponding neoplasm, choroid plexus carcinoma, are seen in the lateral ventricles.

Extra-axial Tumors

Extra-axial tumors include meningiomas (which arise from meninges), neuromas (from the cranial nerves), pituitary, and pineal tumors. Meningiomas are slow growing and well circumscribed, they have a broad dural base, and they contain punctate calcifications. These tumors enhance homogeneously after contrast administration and may be solitary or multiple. The adjacent bone typically demonstrates reactive thickening. Metastases present as multiple brain masses located at the gray-white matter junction, where they get deposited by hematogenous spread. Surrounding edema is seen adjacent to brain neoplasms (low-density, dark on CT and high signal intensity, white on T2).

Posterior Cranial Fossa Tumors

In adults metastatic disease is most common, followed by hemangioblastoma; in children gliomas of the cerebellum occur most frequently. Hemangioblastomas are benign neoplasms of endothelial origin, and their typical appearance is cystic with a brightly enhancing mural nodule. Of interest is the cerebellar and spinal hemangioblastomas' association with von Hippel-Lindau syndrome.

KEY POINTS
1. The best imaging modality for brain neoplasms is MRI with gadolinium enhancement.
2. Contrast-enhanced CT should not be used instead of MRI because its anatomic detail is poor in comparison.
3. PET CT is gaining ground for monitoring brain malignancy recurrence because it can distinguish between the high metabolism of tumor from the metabolically inactive postsurgical changes.
4. MRI spectroscopy is now used to predict a mass as neoplasm versus infection.

■ BRAIN ABSCESS

Anatomy

A **brain abscess** is a collection of pus within the cerebral-cerebellar parenchyma. The necrotic brain tissue becomes encapsulated by glial cells and fibroblasts. A subdural empyema is a collection of pus between the dura mater and the arachnoid and is due to a peripheral abscess rupture into the arachnoid space or direct extension of extracerebral infections.

Etiology

A variety of pathogens are responsible for brain abscesses (anaerobic bacteria, fungi, parasites such as *Taenia solium cysticerci* and protozoa such as *Toxoplasma gondii*).

Epidemiology

Brain abscesses can occur in either immunocompromised or immunocompetent hosts.

Pathogenesis

Brain abscesses occur either as a result of direct extension of other cranial infections (sinusitis, mastoiditis, etc.) or by hematogenous spread of infection (from endocarditis, lung abscess, etc.).

Clinical Manifestations

History

Patients present with headache, fever, chills, seizures, and lethargy.

Physical Examination

The complications are due to mass effect and brain edema, which may lead to brain herniation. Papilledema, anisocoria, and any other focal neurologic deficits should alert the physician of a brain mass (infectious or noninfectious).

Diagnostic Evaluation

Lumbar puncture is contraindicated because the increased intracranial pressure and the organism yield from cerebrospinal fluid (CSF) are relatively low (even when the abscess ruptures). MRI and CT are the radiologic tools for diagnosis.

Radiologic Findings

A "ring-enhancing" lesion CT or MRI is suggestive of the diagnosis. Noncontrast CTs of the brain are routinely ordered, and an area of low density (necrotic center) with a higher attenuation peripherally can thus be visualized (Figure 3-10); the imaging appearance makes it hard to distinguish it from a neoplasm. It is generally believed that tumor peripheral enhancement is more nodular and irregular. The cortical side of an abscess wall is usually thicker because it has better blood supply. An area of edema surrounds an encapsulated infection, but it also surrounds a tumor.

Small adjacent abscesses can form (daughter abscesses). Multiple small ring-enhancing lesions should raise the possibility of toxoplasmosis. Neurocysticercosis is caused by larvae of *Taenia solium* and, in the acute phase of infestation, the ring-enhancing cystic lesions demonstrate the scolex within.

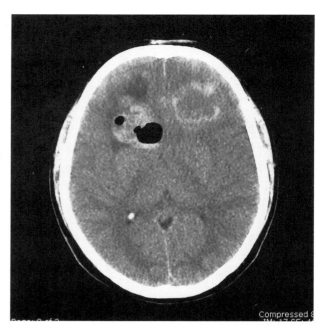

Figure 3-10 • Brain abscesses. Noncontrast CT of the brain demonstrates gas within a brain abscess in the right lower frontal lobe. Note the lower-density area with high attenuation at the periphery in the contralateral left frontal lobe representing a second abscess.
(Courtesy of University of Southern California Medical Center, Los Angeles, CA.)

Treatment

Treatment must be started and must cover a variety of organisms because brain abscesses can be fatal. Stereotactic or open drainage of the abscess may be required if medical treatment response is unsatisfactory or the mass effect and edema are significant. Antiparasitic treatment (albendazole) may be initiated in acute neurocysticercosis to reduce the severity of symptoms (seizures).

KEY POINTS

1. It is sometimes difficult to distinguish between a neoplastic versus infectious mass on the basis of imaging. On contrast-enhanced MRI or CT, both present as ring-enhancing lesions. Use of MRI spectroscopy appears promising.
2. In emergency situations, to obtain a fast preliminary diagnosis, noncontrast CT can be used, but the study of choice is always MRI.

Thoracic Imaging

ANATOMY AND GENERAL PRINCIPLES

The single most common diagnostic imaging examination today remains the chest radiograph. Every physician should develop a systematic approach to reading it. First, the physician confirms the patient's and then the projection of the film. In the posterior-anterior (PA) projection (Figure 4-1A), the patient's chest is closer to the film compared to the anterior-posterior (AP) projection, where the patient's back is closer to the film. In the PA view, the clavicles appear slightly lower on the film, the scapulae project more laterally, and the posterior elements of the vertebral bodies are more clearly visualized than on an AP film. The PA projection is preferred because the heart is closer to the film, it is less magnified, and its size is more accurately displayed. The lateral film (Figure 4-1B) is generally used in conjunction with the PA film and provides more information about cardiac enlargement, pleural effusions, location of lung parenchymal pathology, and the position of mediastinal masses.

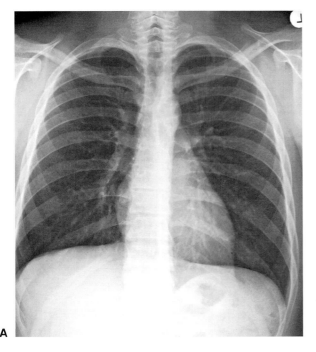

A

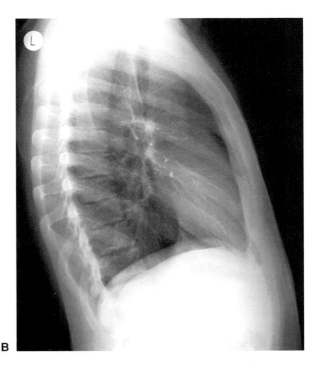

B

Figure 4-1 • **A:** Normal PA chest radiograph. **B:** Normal lateral chest radiograph. **C:** Normal portable AP chest radiograph. (Courtesy of Cedars-Sinai Medical Center, Los Angeles, CA.)

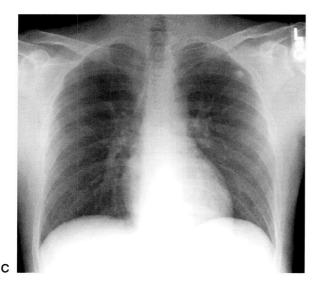

C

Figure 4-1 • Continued

For an adequate PA radiograph, the patient must be able to stand or sit in a wheelchair. If the patient is too unstable or too ill to come to the imaging department for the PA film, an AP radiograph is obtained using a portable x-ray machine (Figure 4-1C). A portable film in supine position usually makes the evaluation of pulmonary parenchyma and of heart size difficult. Patients are usually too ill to take a deep inspiration, and pneumothoraces may be missed (see further discussion in this chapter).

Radiologic Considerations

The next step in reading a chest radiograph is using a systematic approach **(ABCDE)** to evaluate the five essential areas of the film:

1. **A**ir: lungs, including central airways and pulmonary vessels
2. **B**ones: ribs, clavicles, spine, shoulders, and scapulae
3. **C**ardiac: heart and mediastinum
4. **D**iaphragm and pleural surfaces
5. **E**verything else: lines and tubes, upper abdomen, soft tissues of the chest wall and neck

When a systematic approach is used during every examination, nothing on the film will be left uninspected. First, the lungs are normally the darkest portions of the film because the air within the alveoli is easily penetrated by the x-ray beam. The lungs will span about nine or ten posterior ribs or, in normal inspiration, seven to eight anterior ribs. The pulmonary vessels are normally seen radiating from the hila, with

gradual tapering to the periphery. The normal distribution of the pulmonary vessels is two thirds of the blood flow to the lower portions of the lungs and one third to the upper lobes. The lungs are scrutinized for focal areas of abnormality, such as atelectasis, masses, or nodules, and then for diffuse processes, such as alveolar or interstitial patterns. An alveolar or "airspace" pattern is a confluent opacification, often confined to one lobe or lobar segment, as in pneumonia. Air normally found in the alveoli has been replaced by more radio-opaque material, such as pus, water, blood, cells, or proteinaceous material. An interstitial pattern is often described as lace-like or "reticular."

The next area of focus is the skeleton; inspection of the osseous structures was described previously. Particular attention is given to the ribs and spine for fractures and metastatic lesions, and the shoulders are examined for evidence of arthritis.

Evaluation of the cardiac silhouette and mediastinum is crucial for interpretation of the chest radiograph. The mediastinum is divided into anterior, middle, and posterior sections as seen on a lateral chest radiograph. The anterior mediastinum includes the anterior chest wall to the anterior heart border. Pathology that may be found here includes the "four Ts": thyroid masses, thymoma, teratoma, and "terrible lymphoma." The middle mediastinum includes the heart, hilar structures, esophagus, and descending aorta.

Common pathologies in this area include lymph-node enlargement, hiatal hernia, descending aortic aneurysm, and esophageal pathology. The posterior mediastinum on the lateral radiograph includes the thoracic vertebral bodies and paravertebral soft tissues.

In the frontal (PA or AP) projections of the chest, several landmarks of the mediastinum are useful in finding pathology. On the right side of the mediastinum three convexities or "moguls" are located. From superior to inferior, these are the superior vena cava, ascending aorta, and right atrium. Increased soft-tissue volume in the region of the superior vena cava (to the right of the trachea) usually represents abnormally enlarged lymph nodes. On the left margin of the mediastinum, the three convexities are the aortic arch, pulmonary artery outflow tract, and left ventricle. Between the left-sided moguls, there are normally two concavities: the aortopulmonary window and the region of the left atrial appendage. If either of these two concavities is replaced by soft tissue, the mediastinum is abnormal and further workup is required.

When lung pathology is found, an effort should be made to describe its location, including the lobe, and, if possible, the segment. One method of making this determination is to look for areas that are silhouetted or obscured by the pathology. For example, any lesion that obscures the right- or left-side heart border must be in either the right middle lobe or the lingual, respectively. If either hemidiaphragm is silhouetted, the pathology is in the adjacent lower lobe.

Another general principle in reading chest radiographs is making a determination of the predominant pattern in the lungs. Certain patterns may suggest specific diseases, but more often the patterns overlap; that is, granulomatous disease of the lung may mimic metastatic lung nodules. One should also keep in mind the broad categories into which pathologic processes can be classified. One mnemonic is "**MACHINE**": **m**etabolic, **a**utoimmune, **c**ongenital, **h**ematologic, **i**nfectious, **n**eoplastic, and **e**nvironmental. Of course, some pathology will not fit into these groups, but most will, and reviewing the list each time will be helpful in generating a differential diagnosis.

One way to avoid common errors is to avoid the temptation to evaluate a chest film with a "quick glance." Sometimes, when the main finding on the film is discovered, the remainder of the systematic approach is abandoned, and secondary findings may be missed. This type of mistake is commonly referred to as a "satisfaction of search" error.

KEY POINTS

1. The chest radiograph is the most common imaging study.
2. A systematic approach with evaluation of the air, bones, cardiac shadow, diaphragm, and everything else is essential in the interpretation of any chest film.
3. Alveolar opacification of the lungs represents blood, water, or pus in the acute phase and either cells or protein in the chronic stage.
4. When pathology is found, a thorough evaluation of the film is crucial to avoid the "satisfaction of search" error.

INFECTION

■ LOBAR PNEUMONIA

Anatomy

The most common anatomy entails three right and two left pulmonary lobes, but some variations exist.

Etiology

Lobar pneumonia is almost always bacterial. Common pathogens are *Streptococcus pneumoniae*, *Haemophilus influenzae*, *Klebsiella pneumoniae*, and *Neisseria meningitidis*.

Epidemiology

Lobar pneumonia is encountered in both adults and children.

Clinical Manifestations

History

Patients with lobar pneumonia present with chief complaints of fever, productive cough, and shortness of breath. Symptoms generally start gradually and worsen over 2 to 4 days. Some patients complain of chest pain or abdominal pain in some cases of lower-lobe pneumonia.

Physical Examination

Dullness to percussion, egophony, and tactile fremitus are classic physical findings with lobar consolidation. Rales are often heard over the affected segments. If the lung is consolidated and air cannot penetrate into the alveoli, decreased breath sounds are noted.

Diagnostic Evaluation

Usually a single plain film of the chest is used for diagnosis. Sputum cultures are routinely used; in more severe cases, if sputum cultures are not diagnostic or if patients are not responding to therapy, bronchoscopy may be used.

Radiologic Findings

The radiologic appearance of pneumonia varies depending on several factors, including the type of pathogen (whether bacterial, viral, fungal, or atypical), underlying lung disease (chronic obstructive pulmonary disease [COPD], chronic interstitial lung disease, cystic fibrosis), and risk factors for the patient (aspiration risk, immunocompromise, exposure to TB).

Most cases of bacterial pneumonia have the common appearance of alveolar opacification in a lobar distribution on chest radiograph (Figure 4-2). The process may affect an entire lobe and demonstrate a sharp border with the adjacent lobe, or it may only involve specific segments of a lobe. Some radiologists compare the appearance of alveolar opacification to a

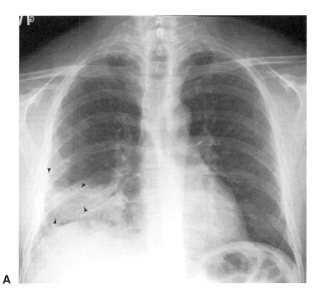

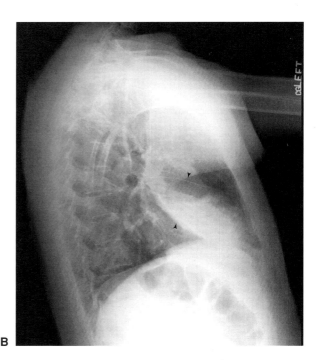

Figure 4-2 • A: Lobar pneumonia on PA chest radiograph. There is alveolar opacification in the lateral segment of the right middle lobe. **B:** Lobar pneumonia. Lateral view in the same patient as (A) with alveolar opacification outlining the borders of the right middle lobe.
(Courtesy of Cedars-Sinai Medical Center, Los Angeles, CA.)

patchy fog overlying the film. Often air bronchograms are seen, which are evident because air remains in the bronchi and is surrounded by densely consolidated adjacent lung tissue, creating an air-tissue interface. The air-tissue interface is evident on the radiograph because of the differences in attenuation (see Figure 4-2). It must be noted, however, that air bronchograms are nonspecific and do not equate exclusively with pneumonia. They only demonstrate that the process is within the lung parenchyma, not in the pleural space or overlying soft tissue. Usually there is little or no associated volume loss with lobar pneumonia because the bronchi are filled with air and do not collapse. It is very important to obtain a follow-up chest x-ray (CXR, at about 6 weeks) to ensure resolution. At times, a neoplasm may mimic pneumonia, or a tumor may cause a postobstructive infection.

■ BRONCHOPNEUMONIA

Anatomy

In contrast to lobar pneumonia, which affects the alveoli, bronchopneumonia affects primarily the bronchi, bronchioles, and some scattered adjacent alveoli.

KEY POINTS

1. Bacterial pneumonia is commonly caused by *S. pneumoniae, H. influenzae, K. pneumoniae,* and *N. meningitidis.*
2. Alveolar opacification in a lobar distribution on chest radiograph is the classic radiographic finding for bacterial pneumonia.
3. Alveolar opacification looks like a patchy fog overlying the film.
4. Air bronchograms are common in lobar pneumonia.

Etiology

Common pathogens include *Staphylococcus aureus,* gram-negatives, and in some cases *Mycoplasma pneumoniae* (which may also present with an interstitial pattern).

Epidemiology

Infants and children are more commonly affected by viruses.

Pathogenesis

The common mechanism of spread is by inhalation of infectious droplets. The bronchi become inflamed and filled with pus and the distal alveoli collapse. The volume loss is appreciated on radiographs.

Clinical Manifestations

History and Physical Examination

Refer to the lobar pneumonia history and examination findings.

Diagnostic Evaluation

Again a CXR is the study of choice. Sputum cultures are used, but their yield is often limited. Bronchoscopy is invasive as the initial study.

Radiologic Findings

Patchy opacification in a segmental as opposed to a lobar distribution is common with bronchopneumonia (Figure 4-3). Air bronchograms are not present as in lobar pneumonia because the bronchi are filled with exudate and there is no air-tissue interface to delineate them.

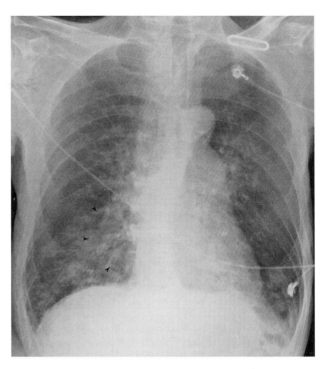

Figure 4-3 • Bronchopneumonia. There is patchy alveolar opacification of the right middle lobe with silhouetting of the right-sided heart border. This 88-year-old patient had silent aspiration on a video swallowing study. The findings represent aspiration pneumonia.
(Courtesy of Cedars-Sinai Medical Center, Los Angeles, CA.)

KEY POINTS

1. Bronchopneumonia causes patchy opacification on chest radiograph because of the collapse of distal alveoli.
2. Air bronchograms are usually not present as with lobar pneumonia.

▇ ASTHMA

Etiology

The bronchoconstrictor response of the asthmatic is exaggerated, but the cause for hyperreactive airways is still not certain.

Epidemiology

A large percentage of population is affected by asthma, African Americans in particular.

Pathogenesis

The pathogenesis of asthma involves hyperreactive airway mucosa, a low threshold for degranulation of mast cells in response to irritants, and increased immunoglobulin E (IgE) levels. As the airway mucosa becomes edematous and spasm of the bronchial smooth muscle occurs, the lumen narrows and the result is decreased air movement. The effect is mostly on the bronchioles and smaller airways, but all central airways may be involved.

Clinical Manifestations

History

Patients complain of shortness of breath, wheezing, and sometimes cough.

Physical Examination

Prolonged expiration, decreased breath sounds, expiratory wheezes, and accessory muscle use for resting respiration are common physical findings.

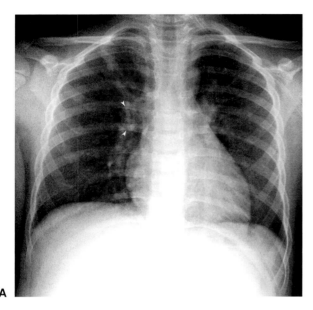

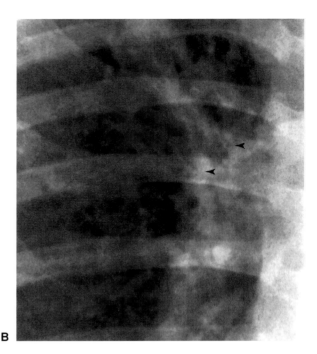

A   **B**

Figure 4-4 • **A:** Asthma. AP chest radiograph demonstrates hyperinflated lungs and peribronchial cuffing or edema surrounding the medium-sized airways. **B:** Asthma. Magnification of right upper lobe bronchi with peribronchial edema.
(Courtesy of Cedars-Sinai Medical Center, Los Angeles, CA.)

Diagnostic Evaluation

A chest x-ray is always obtained.

Radiologic Findings

Radiographically most patients with asthma will have a normal CXR. However, there may be evidence of hyperinflated lungs (Figure 4-4A), atelectasis, and peribronchial cuffing (Figure 4-4B). Hyperinflated lungs are determined by an inspiratory result that demonstrates more than 10 posterior ribs above the diaphragm, often with an increased retrosternal air space seen on the lateral view. Peribronchial cuffing is the radiographic manifestation of edema surrounding the bronchial tree. It is a nonspecific finding that is sometimes seen in other lung processes, such as chronic bronchitis, bronchiec-

tasis, pulmonary edema, and cystic fibrosis. Taking into consideration the patient's past medical history can help in distinguishing these disorders.

■ NEOPLASMS

Anatomy

It is essential to define the location of a lung neoplasm as parenchymal, mediastinal, or pleural based because the clinical presentations, differential diagnoses, and treatments differ for each. Smoking is the greatest risk factor for lung neoplasm, and about 92% of patients with lung cancer have a history of smoking. From another point of view, 10% of all heavy smokers (more than 35 pack-years) will develop lung cancer. The most common type of cancer found in smokers is squamous cell carcinoma, followed by adenocarcinoma. Often lung cancer will metastasize. Common sites of metastases are liver, adrenal glands, distant lung parenchyma, brain, and, less commonly, bone. So a suspected lung tumor warrants at least CT of the chest and abdomen (liver and adrenals should be included) for staging. If bone pain is present, a bone scan should be ordered. Cancers that commonly

---

KEY POINTS

1. Patients with asthma commonly have a normal CXR.
2. Hyperinflated lungs, peribronchial inflammation, and atelectasis are nonspecific, associated radiographic findings with asthma.

metastasize *to* the lungs are breast, renal, colon, testicular, melanomas, and sarcomas.

■ BRONCHOGENIC CARCINOMA

Etiology

The term **bronchogenic carcinoma** is a broad classification that defines a neoplasm that arises within a bronchus but includes several different cell types. Cigarette smoking is considered the main cause for bronchogenic carcinoma (occupational agents are less frequent etiologic factors).

Epidemiology

Examples of bronchogenic lesions include adenocarcinoma (45%), squamous cell carcinoma (35%), small cell carcinoma (15%), and large cell carcinoma (1%–5%).

Clinical Manifestations

History

A history of weight loss and persistent cough is usually elicited. Hemoptysis is relatively common with endobronchial lesions. Some patients may present with chest pain if the chest wall is involved.

Physical Examination

Decreased breath sounds resulting from a malignant pleural effusion are common. Abnormal breath sounds are also present.

Diagnostic Evaluation

A chest x-ray should be obtained. Bronchoscopic or transthoracic biopsy (under CT guidance) can be obtained for cell-type diagnosis. Obtaining cells may be difficult, sometimes requiring invasive procedures (open biopsy or mediastinoscopy). A CT scan should be ordered to stage the cancer (contralateral involvement, liver and adrenal metastases).

Radiologic Findings

The appearance of adenocarcinoma on plain film and CT is that of a peripheral mass (>5 cm) or nodule (<5 cm), often with spiculated borders (Figure 4-5). A subtype of adenocarcinoma, bronchioalveolar carcinoma, has a different radiographic appearance. Bronchioalveolar carcinoma may present as multiple

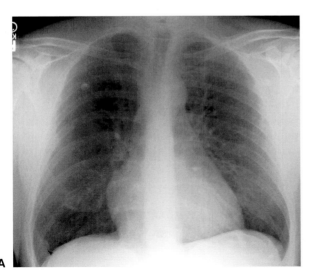

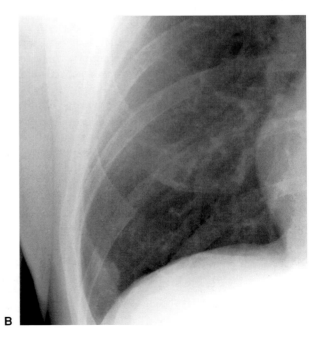

Figure 4-5 • A: Adenocarcinoma of the lung. PA chest radiograph with right lower lobe peripheral nodule near the right costophrenic angle. **B:** Adenocarcinoma of the lung. Magnification of lung nodule in (A) shows subtle, poorly demarcated nodule. **C:** Adenocarcinoma on CT of the chest with lung windows. A spiculated, peripheral soft-tissue mass is seen in the right lower lobe. (Courtesy of Cedars-Sinai Medical Center, Los Angeles, CA.)

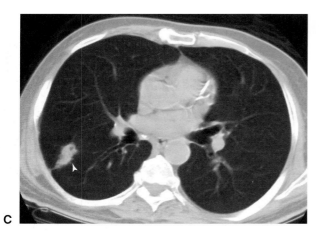

C

Figure 4-5 • Continued

nodules, with chronic airspace consolidation, or as an interstitial pattern as the tumor cells grow along the interstitial framework of the lung producing a "lepidic" or "scale-like" pattern.

Squamous cell carcinoma tends to occur within the walls of a central bronchus and to present with bronchial obstruction and associated atelectasis of the corresponding lobe. Small cell carcinoma also usually presents as a central mass. Large cell carcinoma can be located centrally or peripherally.

A contrast-enhanced CT scan of the chest is the next appropriate test in the assessment of a known pulmonary mass. Today's CT scanners consistently detect nodules as small as 0.3 cm. Associated findings include ipsilateral mediastinal lymphadenopathy, malignant pleural effusions containing neoplastic cells, and atelectasis or postobstructive pneumonia from a lesion that occludes a bronchus. Lymph nodes are best seen using soft-tissue window and level settings and are considered pathologic if they are larger than 1 cm in the shortest axis. A different appearance is seen with bronchioalveolar carcinoma, which may have a chronic airspace consolidation pattern similar to common pneumonia. Cavitation of a lesion is most commonly seen with squamous cell carcinoma and may help in distinguishing it from the other causes of neoplastic masses.

■ METASTASES

Anatomy

Spread of tumor to lungs is usually to the more vascularized parenchyma, the lung bases.

Etiology

Common sources of hematogenous spread are vascular neoplasms such as renal cell carcinoma, thyroid carcinoma, melanoma, and sarcomas. Common neoplasms that exhibit lymphatic spread are breast, gastric, pancreatic, laryngeal, and cervical carcinomas.

Epidemiology

Both sexes are nearly equally affected.

Pathogenesis

Primary cancers from extrapulmonary sources may metastasize to the lungs by two main mechanisms: **hematogenous spread** through the systemic circulation via the pulmonary arterial blood supply and **lymphatic spread** via the periaortic and celiac lymph nodes to the posterior mediastinal lymph nodes.

Clinical Manifestations

History and Physical Examination

Refer to primary lung tumor history and examination findings.

Diagnostic Evaluation

If cells are obtained by bronchoscopy or transthoracic biopsy, computerized tomography can be ordered to

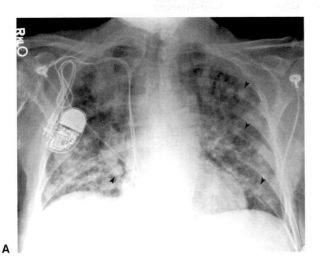

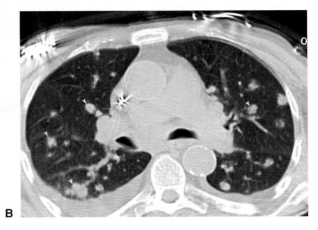

Figure 4-6 • A: Lung metastases. AP chest radiograph with numerous round, well-demarcated metastatic nodules. **B:** Lung metastases. CT scan of the same patient demonstrating numerous metastatic nodules.
(Courtesy of Cedars-Sinai Medical Center, Los Angeles, CA.)

locate the primary tumor. GI tumors may not be identified by CT, so endoscopy should be performed.

Radiologic Findings

Almost exclusively, hematogenous lung metastases appear as multiple variably sized lesions with sharp, round margins (Figure 4-6). They have a propensity for the lung bases more than for the apices because of the relative increase in blood flow in the bases. Metastases from lymphatic spread have a higher percentage of solitary mass lesions at presentation, but they may also have multiple discrete nodules. Associated mediastinal lymphadenopathy is common with both hematogenous and lymphatic metastatic neoplasms.

KEY POINTS

1. Renal cell carcinoma, thyroid carcinoma, melanoma, and sarcomas commonly metastasize to the lungs by hematogenous spread.
2. The classic radiographic appearance of lung metastases is multiple well-demarcated pulmonary nodules.

▮ SARCOIDOSIS

Etiology

Sarcoidosis is a chronic multisystem, granulomatous disease of uncertain etiology.

Epidemiology

The disease is 10 to 20 times more common in blacks than whites and usually occurs in the third to fifth decades of life.

Clinical Manifestations

History

Patients with pulmonary involvement usually present with a cough or with dyspnea. The lung is involved to some degree in about 90% of cases.

Physical Examination

Peripheral lymphadenopathy may be discovered. Some patients present with erythema nodosum, lacrimal gland enlargement, and polyarticular inflammation.

Diagnostic Evaluation

CXR is recommended for detection of mediastinal lymph-node enlargement. Biopsy is needed for confirmation. Angiotensin-converting enzyme (ACE) serum levels should also be drawn.

Radiologic Findings

Radiographically, pulmonary sarcoidosis appears in stages. **Stage 0** occurs before there is radiographic evidence of the disease in an essentially normal film. The diagnosis of sarcoidosis may be made based on involve-

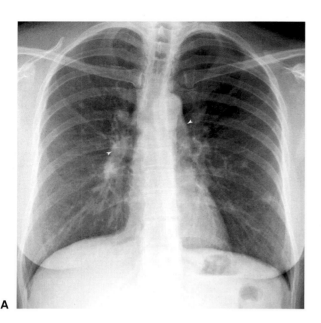
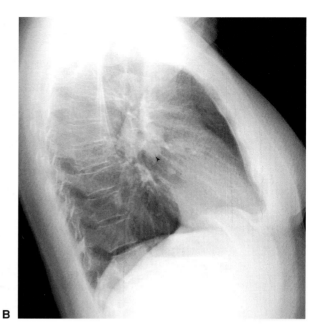

A   **B**

Figure 4-7 • **A:** Sarcoidosis. Bilateral hilar lymph-node enlargement on PA chest radiograph. **B:** Sarcoidosis. Lateral view of the chest with hilar lymph-node enlargement. Compare with normal chest in Figure 4-1B.
(Courtesy of Cedars-Sinai Medical Center, Los Angeles, CA.)

ment of other organs, such as the skin, eyes, liver, or spleen. Hepatosplenomegaly is found in 15% to 20% of all cases. Only 10% of patients will present with stage 0. **Stage 1** pulmonary sarcoidosis demonstrates bilateral symmetric hilar lymphadenopathy and represents 50% of cases (Figure 4-7). Patients present with a nonproductive cough; the adenopathy initiates a cough reflex. **Stage 2** sarcoidosis has bilateral hilar lymphadenopathy, but it also demonstrates reticulonodular parenchymal opacities. Some nodules may reach 1 cm in size, and the initial pattern may progress to appear as patchy consolidation with air bronchograms. As the disease progresses, **stage 3** sarcoidosis involves increased pulmonary parenchymal opacities, but the lymphadenopathy decreases. It is as though the disease process moves out of the hilar lymph nodes into the lungs. **Stage 4** represents end-stage disease with pulmonary fibrosis and bullae formation with upper-lobe predominance.

Chest radiographs are useful for initial diagnosis and monitoring treatment. Chest CT is best for defining the extent of lymphadenopathy at stage 1 and for early detection of progression to stage 2 with interstitial disease. High-resolution CT is useful during stage 2 sarcoidosis because interstitial disease is more evident compared with standard CT imaging of the chest. A nuclear medicine gallium scan will demonstrate increased uptake in the hilar lymph nodes during active

stage 1 disease. It is less sensitive once the process has moved from the hila to the lung parenchyma.

KEY POINTS

1. Sarcoidosis is a chronic granulomatous disease.
2. Bilateral hilar lymph-node enlargement is the classic, though nonspecific, early radiographic finding.
3. Sarcoidosis may progress to involve the lung parenchyma to cause interstitial fibrosis in stage 4 disease.

■ CARDIOMEGALY

Anatomy

When one is looking at a PA chest radiograph, it is common to measure the apparent diameter of the heart and compare it with the span of the chest at the level of the dome of the right hemidiaphragm. If this ratio is greater than half, the cardiac silhouette is enlarged (Figure 4-8). The term **cardiac silhouette** includes the contribution of the pericardium, not just the heart itself. If a large pericardial effusion is present, the cardiac silhouette will appear enlarged even if the heart itself is of normal size. It would be incorrect to

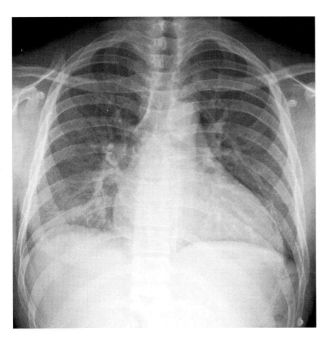

Figure 4-8 • Cardiomegaly. PA chest radiograph demonstrating enlargement of the cardiac silhouette, which spans more than one half the diameter of the chest.
(Courtesy of Cedars-Sinai Medical Center, Los Angeles, CA.)

Clinical Manifestations

History

Cardiomegaly is a finding on an x-ray. If congestive heart failure ensues, then a history of dyspnea on exertion, orthopnea, ankle edema, etc., can be elicited.

Physical Examination

In many cases, the physical examination is normal. The heart apex may be displaced laterally. Signs of heart failure are decreased breath sounds (pleural effusions), wheezing, and pitting ankle edema.

Diagnostic Evaluation

The PA film is more useful than the AP radiograph for determining cardiomegaly because the heart is closer to the film and its size is more accurate with the PA film. A lateral radiograph will yield information as to specific chamber enlargement (Figure 4-9).

Radiologic Findings

The left atrium sits posteriorly on the lateral view and, if it is enlarged, may be seen to bulge toward the

use the term **cardiomegaly** in this case. Measurement of the cardiac silhouette is not accurate on the portable AP radiograph because there is a magnification effect from the heart's increased distance from the film. The cardiac silhouette will always appear slightly larger on an AP film than it truly measures.

Etiology

Causes of an enlarged cardiac silhouette, and more specifically cardiomegaly, include ischemic cardiomyopathy, hypertension, valvular disease, congenital heart disease, and several other less common conditions, such as viral cardiomyopathy and cardiac mass lesions.

Pathogenesis

By far the most common cause of cardiomegaly is ischemic cardiomyopathy, or congestive heart failure, the inability of the heart muscle to keep pace with forward blood flow, in other words, pump failure. This occurs when the cardiac muscle is "stunned" by an acute ischemic event following a myocardial infarct, or it may occur later when there is decreased wall motion in the territory of a coronary artery with a stenosis or occlusion.

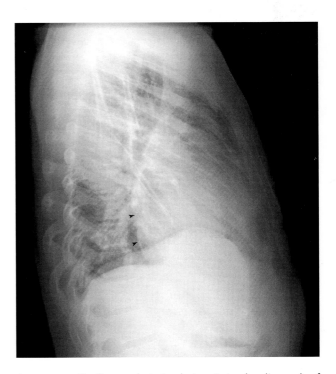

Figure 4-9 • Cardiomegaly. Lateral view. Lateral radiograph of the patient in Figure 4-8 demonstrates cardiomegaly with enlargement of the left atrium; the posterior border of the heart nearly reaches the spine.
(Courtesy of Cedars-Sinai Medical Center, Los Angeles, CA.)

spine. Left ventricular enlargement appears as a rounded left cardiac border with downward displacement of the cardiac apex on the PA view.

■ PULMONARY EDEMA

Etiology

Pulmonary edema occurs in a variety of processes. Most commonly, it is seen with left-sided heart failure, aortic stenosis, and renal failure with total body fluid overload. Another less common category is lung injury that includes adult respiratory distress syndrome (ARDS), sepsis, aspiration, and inhalation injuries.

Clinical Manifestations

History

Patients experience shortness of breath, fatigue, swelling of the lower extremities, and orthopnea.

Physical Examination

On examination, pitting edema in the calves, diminished breath sounds due to pleural effusions, or crackles can all be present.

Diagnostic Evaluation

A chest x-ray, along with an echocardiogram, should be obtained in all patients.

Radiologic Findings

Radiographic features of cardiogenic pulmonary edema can be graded according to severity. **Grade 1** demonstrates upper lung pulmonary vascular congestion where the normal distribution of pulmonary venous blood flow of one third to upper lobes and two thirds to lower lobes is altered. In most cases, the

distribution becomes more half and half as evidenced by increased diameter of the upper lobe pulmonary veins. In **grade 2** cardiogenic pulmonary edema, the radiograph shows peribronchial cuffing, pleural effusions, and Kerley B lines, which represent interstitial edema. **Grade 3** edema has the addition of alveolar opacification, especially in the lung bases and perihilar region (Figure 4-10). Air bronchograms may be seen because the alveoli are filled with water and the bronchi contain air, causing an air-water interface. Decompensated aortic stenosis has similar findings in the setting of cardiac enlargement and elevated left atrial pressures measured with a Swan-Ganz catheter.

Noncardiogenic pulmonary edema is most often associated with renal failure and volume overload. It is common with patients on dialysis. The radiographic appearance is different from cardiogenic pulmonary edema in several ways. First, the heart size is usually normal unless there is also a cardiac comorbidity. Next, the alveolar opacification usually occurs centrally in a perihilar distribution, and air bronchograms are infrequently seen. The pulmonary venous blood flow is usually balanced 50% to each of the upper and lower lung zones. As with cardiogenic edema, pleural effusions and Kerley B lines are common.

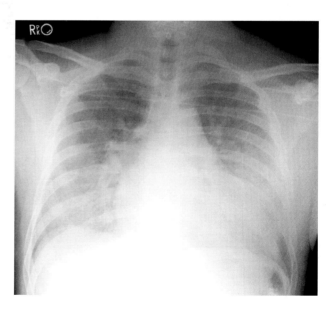

Figure 4-10 • Pulmonary edema. The cardiac silhouette is mildly enlarged, and its borders are not well defined because of the overlying alveolar opacification from edema. The patient had a massive myocardial infarction and flash pulmonary edema. (Courtesy of Cedars-Sinai Medical Center, Los Angeles, CA.)

Edema caused by pulmonary injury predominantly involves the alveoli. It is difficult to distinguish from noncardiogenic pulmonary edema. As a reaction to the initial insult, the alveoli fill with fluid and exudate, causing patchy opacifications and air bronchograms. The heart size and pulmonary vessels are normal, and Kerley B lines and pleural effusions are rarely seen.

KEY POINTS

1. Pulmonary edema is most commonly seen with left-sided heart failure, aortic stenosis, and renal failure with total body fluid overload.
2. Upper-lung pulmonary vascular congestion is the earliest radiographic sign of pulmonary edema.
3. Kerley B lines, peribronchial fluid, and pleural effusions are classic signs of pulmonary vascular congestion and edema.
4. Alveolar opacification represents advanced pulmonary vascular congestion and defines true pulmonary edema.

■ PLEURAL EFFUSION

Anatomy

A pleural effusion represents an increase above the normal physiologic amount of fluid in the pleural space between the parietal and visceral pleura.

Etiology

Pleural effusion is nonspecific and can be associated with many different pathologic processes. The most common causes are cardiogenic and noncardiogenic pulmonary edema, pneumonia, neoplasm, and autoimmune diseases.

Pathogenesis

The two categories of effusions are transudative and exudative. **Transudative effusions** are generally associated with congestive heart failure, cirrhosis, or protein-losing nephropathy. Exudative effusions are commonly associated with neoplastic processes and pneumonia.

Clinical Manifestations

History

Many patients have pleuritic chest pain or dyspnea. Not uncommonly, pleural effusions are detected incidentally on CXR.

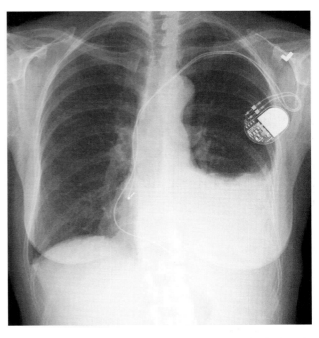

Figure 4-11 • Pleural effusion. PA chest radiograph showing a moderate-sized left pleural effusion, which effaces the left costophrenic angle and left diaphragm.
(Courtesy of Cedars-Sinai Medical Center, Los Angeles, CA.)

Physical Examination

Decreased thoracic excursion, asymmetry of amplitude of hemithoraces, and decreased or absent breath sounds have all been described.

Diagnostic Evaluation

The initial chest x-ray may reveal the cause of pleural effusion (such as pneumonia). To determine whether the effusion is loculated or not, a lateral decubitus x-ray should be ordered. A CT scan of the chest will reveal the size of a pleural effusion (Figure 4-11); it may identify loculations as separate, water-attenuation collections that do not layer along the dependent portion of the chest; and it can distinguish pleural fluid from an adjacent parenchymal process, such as atelectasis or pneumonia.

Radiologic Findings

The radiographic features of a pleural effusion are "blunting" of the costophrenic angles on PA (Figure 4-12) and lateral (Figure 4-13) radiographs, fluid in the horizontal or minor fissures, or thickened pleura

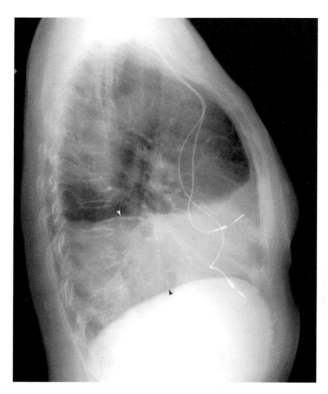

Figure 4-12 • Pleural effusion, lateral view. *White arrowhead* shows top of pleural effusion. *Black arrowhead* is the contralateral (right) hemidiaphragm. The left hemidiaphragm is silhouetted by the pleural fluid.
(Courtesy of Cedars-Sinai Medical Center, Los Angeles, CA.)

laterally or apically on an AP radiograph in a patient positioned more supine than upright or sitting. Lateral decubitus plain films are useful in determining whether the effusion is mobile and therefore can be aspirated during a thoracentesis. The layering pleural effusion on a lateral decubitus film more than 1 cm thick is usually considered of sufficient quantity for thoracentesis.

Occasionally the costophrenic angle appears normal, but an effusion may still be present. This is referred to as a **subpulmonic** effusion and is characterized by fluid that lies between the inferior portion of the lung and the hemidiaphragm. A hint that there is a subpulmonic effusion is that the apex of the hemidiaphragm will appear to be located more lateral than normal on a PA film.

KEY POINTS

1. A pleural effusion is an increase above the normal physiologic amount of fluid in the pleural space between the parietal and visceral pleura.
2. The classic radiographic finding of a pleural effusion is "blunting" of the costophrenic angle, best seen on the lateral view.
3. Lateral decubitus plain films are useful to determine whether the effusion is mobile or loculated.

CHEST TRAUMA

Thoracic injury is thought to account for about 25% of traumatic deaths. A variety of consequences of acute chest trauma, besides the ones touched on in the following paragraphs, is known (e.g., cardiac injury, diaphragm rupture, lung contusion, and laceration). A CXR is nearly always obtained as an initial screening in trauma involving the torso. For the patient with severe trauma, when high clinical suspicion exists for internal-organ injury, a CT scan of the chest with intravenous contrast is obtained. The intravenous contrast is necessary to evaluate the large vessels and to better delineate mediastinal structures (i.e., to facilitate visualization of a mediastinal hematoma).

Radiologic Considerations

Several important clues to diagnosis should be sought for on an initial CXR: gas within the pleural cavity (PTX), mediastinal widening (mediastinal hematoma with or without rupture of the thoracic aorta), and

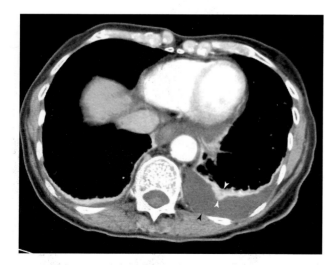

Figure 4-13 • Pleural effusion. CT scan of the chest with soft-tissue windowing. There is a small left pleural effusion *(black arrowhead)* and adjacent atelectasis *(white arrowheads)*.
(Courtesy of Cedars-Sinai Medical Center, Los Angeles, CA.)

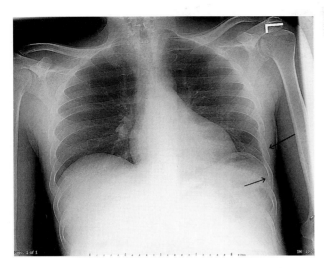

Figure 4-14 • Rib fractures. *Arrows* point to easily missed (by their location) left lateral eighth and ninth rib fractures (note the cortical step off when following each rib).
(Courtesy of University of Southern California Medical Center, Los Angeles, CA.)

chest-wall gas (emphysema). Bones should not be overlooked because fractures and dislocations are common (with the current use of digital radiography, the windowing can be adjusted so the contrast would facilitate identification of rib and vertebral fractures). Particular attention should be given to examining for rib fractures located laterally because these can be easily overlooked (Figure 4-14).

■ PNEUMOTHORAX

Etiology

Gas within the pleural space is common and is due to blunt or penetrating chest trauma.

Pathogenesis

Gas penetrates into the pleural cavity either by penetrating trauma (rib fractures or sharp objects lacerating the parietal pleura) or blunt trauma (tear of bronchi of pulmonary parenchyma).

Clinical Manifestations

History

Eliciting a history may be difficult in the setting of acute trauma. Shortness of breath is common.

Physical Examination

Lack of breath sounds over one hemithorax is a good indication unless a large pleural effusion or hemothorax is present.

Diagnostic Evaluation

Although often limited by technique (portable supine, on a backboard), a CXR is a good start in posttrauma evaluation.

Radiologic Findings

With the patient in the supine position, a smaller pneumothorax can be occult because gas will accumulate anteriorly, layering over the lung. The only clue may be a deepened costophrenic angle on the side of the PTX or the presence of chest-wall emphysema over rib fractures (gas escaping into soft tissues). If it is safe to turn the patient in a lateral decubitus position (but not to place him or her upright), a CXR with the suspected PTX side located nondependently (to allow gas to rise in the pleural cavity in the lateral aspect) can be obtained. If the patient is able to stand, an upright CXR would show a small lucency at the lung apex paralleling the chest wall, located peripherally, and contiguous with a white line (visceral pleura). On an upright CXR, a horizontal air-fluid level signifies a hydropneumothorax (or hemopneumothorax), in contrast to only pleural fluid that has a meniscal configuration (concave at edges).

A small traumatic PTX can be of little clinical consequence, but special precautions should be taken if the patient is intubated because the pressure of air

KEY POINTS

1. A small to moderate-sized pneumothorax can be observed with serial x-rays, without intervention, if the patient is not in critical condition. Assisted ventilation increases the risk of enlarging the volume of gas in the pleural space and can create a tension pneumothorax (leading to circulatory compromise and death).
2. With the patient in the supine position, a pneumothorax can be missed because air layers anteriorly along the chest wall and the x-ray is oriented perpendicularly to the air-lung interface. A deepened costophrenic angle may be the only sign.

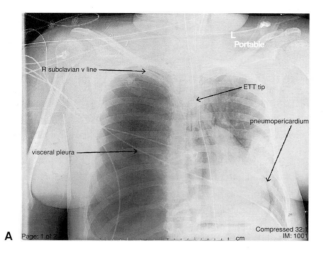

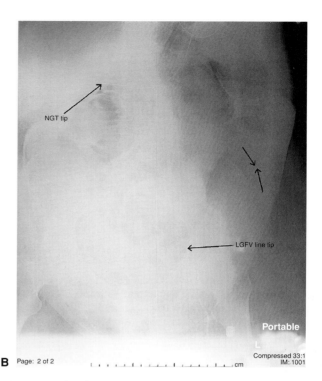

Figure 4-15 • A: Tension pneumothorax. Placement of a right subclavian venous line lead to a pneumothorax, severely enlarged by the assisted ventilation. Note the mediastinal shift with leftward displacement of the nasogastric tube (NGT) and endotracheal tube (ETT). Gas is also present in the pericardial space (pneumopericardium). **B:** The air from the tension pneumothorax dissected into the peritoneum. *Arrows* point to the abnormally seen both sides of the colon wall outlined by the extraluminal gas. (Courtesy of University of Southern California Medical Center, Los Angeles, CA.)

delivered by the ventilator can rapidly enlarge a pneumothorax. As air accumulates within the pleural space, and no exit is provided (a chest tube), a tension PTX is created (life-threatening as the high chest pressure prevents blood return to the heart) and hypotension ensues. A tension PTX is suggested on CXR by a mediastinal shift to the contralateral side and caudad displacement of the ipsilateral diaphragm. The gas can eventually escape the chest cavity by dissecting through planes into the abdomen (intraperitoneally and retroperitoneally) and neck (Figure 4-15).

■ AORTIC RUPTURE

Anatomy

The most common aortic rupture site is at the root of the aorta, but patients with this condition do not survive to the emergency room. The aortic transections diagnosed in the emergency department are those located just proximal to the ligamentum arteriosum or, less frequently, at the diaphragmatic hiatus.

Etiology

Aortic rupture is not uncommon in high-speed motor-vehicle collisions and is the result of shearing forces (rapid deceleration). A high mortality rate occurs with this injury (nearly 90%); most patients exsanguinate before reaching a hospital.

Pathogenesis

The aortic transection occurs due to rapid deceleration forces.

Clinical Manifestations

History

The history of high-velocity motor-vehicle accident should alert the clinician to the possibility of aortic laceration.

Physical Examination

A contained aortic transection (a lumen is maintained by the adjacent connective tissue) may be asymptomatic. Severe hypotension signals blood extravasation out of the lumen.

Diagnostic Evaluation

With chest trauma, an initial CXR is always obtained. A CT scan should also be ordered if suspicion is high and the patient is stable. The definitive diagnostic tool is conventional angiography, which is used for better anatomy delineation or in cases in which the CT scan is negative, but the clinical suspicion still warrants further investigation.

Radiologic Findings

Widening of the mediastinum on a CXR should augment clinical suspicion. Of course other causes of mediastinal prominence exist (e.g., aortic aneurysms, enlarged lymph nodes), but in the clinical setting of trauma, aortic rupture should be the first in the differential. A left apical pleural hemothorax is infrequent, but it is consistent with an aortic tear. Many other x-ray correlations have been made, but they all lack sensitivity and specificity. A CT scan can show the aortic wall irregularity (Figures 4-16 and 4-17), the extrava-

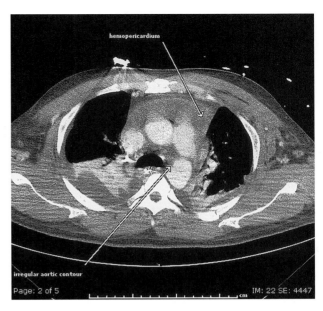

Figure 4-17 • Aortic laceration. Note the irregular descending aorta contour (instead of a normal circular configuration) and the resultant hemopericardium.
(Courtesy of University of Southern California Medical Center, Los Angeles, CA.)

sation of contrast at the rupture site, or a mediastinal hematoma (blood within the mediastinum, which can also be due to benign tears of small veins).

If high clinical suspicion exists, even without definite findings on CT, a conventional thoracic aortogram (see Chapter 10) or a CT angiogram can be obtained to delineate the aorta and site of injury clearly. The CT angiogram is a CT that is timed so the injection of contrast maximally opacifies the aorta and is obtained with thin slices that permit reconstruction of the vessel in different planes.

Treatment

Open vascular surgical repair and endoluminal interventional radiology repair of aortic transection are the

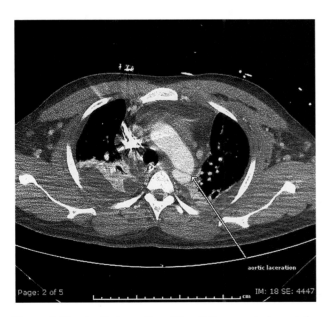

Figure 4-16 • Aortic laceration. CT soft-tissues window at the level of the aortic arch shows a low-density line just posterior to the arch (arrow). The same image also demonstrates bilateral pleural effusions (low-density fluid in the dependent pleural space of the chest) and compressive changes of the underlying lung (high density), which are worse on the right.
(Courtesy of University of Southern California Medical Center, Los Angeles, CA.)

KEY POINTS

1. Aortic injury can be diagnosed by computerized tomography (best by computerized tomography angiogram), but, if a high clinical suspicion exists, a conventional angiogram should be performed,
2. Aortic lacerations can now be treated endovascularly by placing a stent graft to cover the injury site.

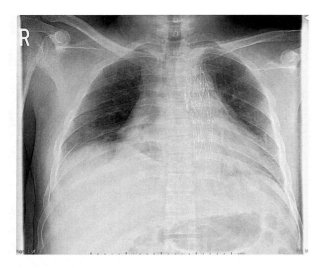

Figure 4-18 • Aortic stent deployed at the site of traumatic aortic rupture in the patient on previous image. CXR is taken after endoluminal repair (done by a vascular interventional radiologist) of the thoracic aortic injury.
(Courtesy of University of Southern California Medical Center, Los Angeles, CA.)

two treatments of choice. The endoluminal approach is obviously chosen when a patient is not believed to be in a condition that would permit an open surgical approach. The intervenional radiologist introduces an aortic stent through the common femoral artery and deploys it at the site of rupture under fluoroscopic guidance (Figure 4-18).

■ PULMONARY THROMBOEMBOLISM

A large pulmonary embolus (PE) is a life-threatening event that can result in sudden death from obstruction of lung parenchyma perfusion, and this condition must be diagnosed promptly for treatment to be instituted. PEs may be acute or chronic.

Anatomy

The lungs are supplied dually: by the pulmonary arterial circulation and by the systemic bronchial arteries. The dual circulation and abundant anastomoses at the terminal bronchioles make lung infarct a relatively unusual occurrence in healthy individuals. Two left and one right bronchial artery usually exist. The pulmonary trunk branches into right and left pulmonary arteries. Before these two arteries enter the pulmonary hila, they each give off a branch to the superior lobe. The pulmonary arteries further divide to supply each pulmonary lobe, bronchopulmonary segment, and lobule. The emboli often lodge at the pulmonary arterial bifurcations. The ones seated at a large arterial bifurcation have been termed **saddle emboli**. In long-standing pulmonary artery occlusion, affected lung segments can maintain perfusion by collaterals from bronchial arteries without developing overt infarcts.

Etiology

PE is most commonly a consequence of deep venous thrombosis, whereas thrombosis in situ, amniotic fluid, fat (post fracture or orthopedic surgery), and air emboli are rarer.

Pathogenesis

The consequences of PE depend on the patient's overall health, ranging from severe pulmonary hypertension with cor pulmonale and shock to mild impairment of pulmonary circulation with preservation of ventilation to the affected lung.

Clinical Manifestations

History
Patients relate a variety of symptoms: from shortness of breath and pleuritic chest pain (i.e., pain on deep inspiration caused by blood deprivation of the pleura) to vague complaints (i.e., near-syncope episode). Clinicians are usually clued in to the diagnosis by the patient's risk factors (e.g., cancer, pregnancy, prolonged immobility, recent surgery, or traveling).

Physical Examination
No specific physical findings are described. In cases in which pulmonary infarction has also developed, pulmonary signs can be present (wheezing, pleural friction rub).

Diagnostic Evaluation

Because no serum test is reliable (D-dimer-fibrin split products may only suggest absence of thromboembolic disease, if normal), diagnostic radiology is the only confirmatory measure.

The CXR is nearly always normal in PE (unless other concurrent pathology is present) because pulmonary infarcts are rare (see the preceding discussion). In these rare cases a wedge-shaped opacity at the lung periphery has the base abutting the pleural surface.

The V/Q scan is a nuclear medicine modality with a somewhat lower patient radiation exposure than CT, so it is preferred in pregnant patients. If a patient has renal insufficiency but is not on dialysis (intravenous contrast can be cleared from the circulation by dialysis), a V/Q scan is preferred to spare the burden of iodinated contrast on renal function. For details on V/Q scan, refer to Chapter 11.

Some physicians prefer the clear visualization of clot within the pulmonary arteries by CT over the inference of pathology by V/Q scan (Figures 4-19 and 4-20). Also, if concomitant lung pathology is present (e.g., infiltrates, pleural effusions), a V/Q scan will be more difficult to interpret. CT scanning is timed so the intravenous iodinated contrast is most concentrated within the pulmonary arteries (CT pulmonary angiogram). Thin slices are obtained through the chest (usually from the top of the aortic arch to lung bases). Some institutions also use delayed-phase acquisition of data (for venous opacification) with widely spaced images through the abdomen, pelvis, and thighs to evaluate the IVC and the iliac, femoral, and popliteal veins. The venous-phase images are of

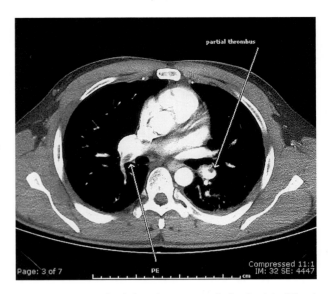

Figure 4-20 • PE. The left pulmonary embolus in this CT pulmonary angiogram causes only partial obliteration of the arterial lumen, and the right one obliterates a segmental branch of the right pulmonary artery.
(Courtesy of University of Southern California Medical Center, Los Angeles, CA.)

limited accuracy because images are not contiguous. So if deep vein thrombosis (DVT) is suspected, an ultrasound of the lower extremities should also be obtained.

If the preceding modalities give an equivocal reading, and it is imperative to have a definite answer, the "gold standard" for diagnosis of PE is still conventional pulmonary angiography. A catheter is introduced by an interventional radiologist under fluoroscopic guidance into the common femoral vein, through the IVC into the right atrium, across the tricuspid valve, and into the pulmonary arteries. Iodinated contrast is injected through the catheter to opacify the pulmonary arteries, and serial x-rays are taken to demonstrate any filling defects within the arteries. This modality is not performed frequently because it is invasive.

Radiologic Findings

By CT or angiogram, chronic PEs manifest as peripheral filling defects adherent to the walls of pulmonary arteries (as lysis and recannalization of the clot occur) or as a smooth cutoff within a pulmonary artery. Acute PEs have an abrupt transition from contrast-opacified vessel to nonopacified arterial lumen.

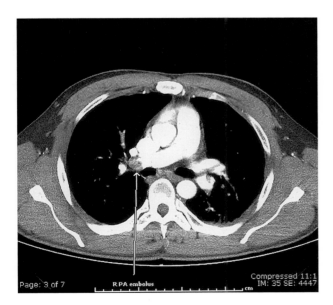

Figure 4-19 • PE. CT pulmonary angiogram with mediastinal windowing demonstrates a large filling defect within the right pulmonary artery *(arrow)*.
(Courtesy of University of Southern California Medical Center, Los Angeles, CA.)

KEY POINTS

1. Pulmonary thromboembolism can manifest as sudden death or mild shortness of breath, or tachycardia, or it may be an incidental finding on CT.
2. Starting treatment early for large emboli is important to preserve lung circulation and to prevent cardiac effects.
3. Emboli lodge within the pulmonary arteries, usually at bifurcations, and infarction is usually prevented by collaterals from the bronchial arteries.

■ SMALL-BOWEL OBSTRUCTION

Anatomy

The small bowel is divided into three main segments: the duodenum, jejunum, and ileum. On a kidneys, ureters, and bladder radiograph (KUB), the small bowel is sometimes seen as scattered gas bubbles throughout the abdomen. Each segment of the small bowel has a general location that helps to distinguish it from the large bowel. The duodenum is the portion of intestine that forms a C-loop in the mid and right upper abdomen and is divided into four segments from the duodenal bulb to the ligament of Treitz. The jejunum is a long segment of intestine coiled in the left upper abdomen that has thin, circular folds called valvulae conniventes. These folds help to distinguish small bowel from large bowel, which have thicker, incomplete folds, called **haustra.** The ileum, located mostly in the mid and right lower abdomen, also has valvulae conniventes. It is the terminal portion of the small intestine and is responsible for the absorption of bile salts and fat-soluble vitamins A, D, E, K, and of vitamin B_{12}.

Etiology

A small-bowel obstruction is defined as an interruption of the normal antegrade transit of intestinal contents. Obstructions are mechanical in nature; that is, the force of antegrade flow is lower than that needed to move intestinal material through the point of obstruction. Obstructions may be partial, allowing some passage of intestinal contents, or they may be complete. One of the most common causes is the formation of adhesions that form scarlike bands and constrict a portion of bowel. Adhesions sometimes occur after intra-abdominal surgery or in areas of prior inflammation. The second most common cause of small-bowel obstruction is hernia. The two main classifications of hernia are abdominal wall and internal. Other causes of small-bowel obstruction include neoplasm, intussusception, ischemia, volvulus, Crohn disease, Meckel diverticulum, gallstone ileus (a clue to which is gas within the biliary tree, seen on plain radiographs or on CT), and intramural hematoma.

Epidemiology

Patients who have had prior intra-abdominal surgery are at increased risk for obstruction from the formation of adhesions. A hernia or intraluminal bowel mass may also be a lead point for obstruction. Any intra-abdominal neoplasm (e.g., lymphoma) may encase bowel, leading to obstruction. Crohn disease with stricture formation is a risk factor.

Clinical Manifestations

History

Patients present with abdominal pain, nausea, vomiting, and obstipation. Pain is often diffuse and crampy, occurring as peristalsis pushes against the obstruction at intervals of 5 to 15 minutes. Nausea and vomiting are most common in proximal small-bowel obstruction because the stomach and duodenum dilate early. Obstipation occurs when intestinal material does not pass into the colon. The fecal material present at the time of the obstruction may pass, but lack of flatus and bowel movements is an important portion of the history.

Physical Examination

An essential portion of the physical examination is the presence of high-pitched, "tinkling" bowel sounds as intestinal contents attempt to squeeze through a narrowed lumen. Abdominal distension is often seen as a late finding as small bowel loops fill with gas and fluid. The abdomen may be tympanitic to percussion as a result of gaseous distension.

Diagnostic Evaluation

The first test to order in suspected small-bowel obstruction is the acute abdominal series, which consists of three films: an upright chest x-ray, an upright KUB (Figure 5-1A) and a supine KUB (Figure 5-1B). The difference between a KUB and an abdominal plain film is the position of the film over the abdomen. The KUB, as its name implies, is a radiograph that includes the kidneys, ureters, and bladder. The abdominal plain film visualizes the top of the diaphragm and does not include as much of the lower abdomen as the KUB, usually only to the level of the iliac crests. Bowel obstruction may also be diagnosed with a CT of the abdomen in patients who experience abdominal pain (Figure 5-2). CT often demonstrates the site of obstruction as well as inflammation or neoplastic involvement. Oral contrast is preferable but not absolutely necessary. A small-bowel series with oral contrast is often performed in an attempt to elucidate the point of obstruction, but these examinations often take several hours because of the delayed transit time through the obstructed intestine, and they are of limited value.

Radiologic Findings

The acute abdominal series often has air-fluid levels on the upright KUB (see Figure 5-1A) and dilated loops of small bowel on the supine KUB (see Figure 5-1B). Small bowel is differentiated from colon by its valvulae conniventes or plica circulares. These are the transverse folds that completely encircle the small bowel as opposed to the colonic haustra, which only cover about half the transverse distance across a given segment of colon. The exclusion of free gas under the diaphragm on the chest radiograph is important because its presence indicates a perforated viscus. If biliary gas is seen centrally within the liver, it is usually the result of prior biliary surgery; although gallstone ileus is also a rare consideration. If portal venous gas is seen at the periphery of the liver, ischemic bowel should be high on the differential diagnosis. The presence of ascites increases the concern for bowel perforation, underlying malignancy, or peritonitis.

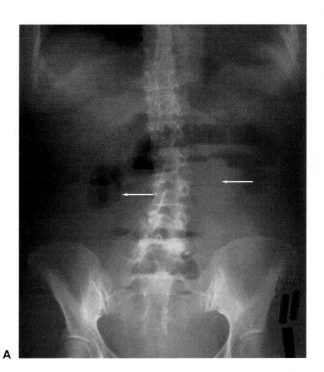

A

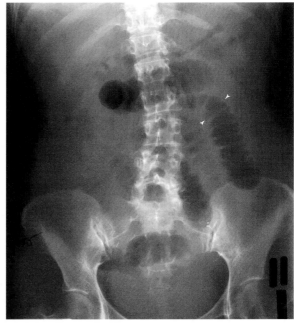

B

Figure 5-1 • Small-bowel obstruction. Upright **(A)** and supine **(B)** KUB films demonstrate dilated air-filled loops of small bowel on the supine film and air-fluid levels on the upright film. This 60-year-old woman has a history of abdominal surgery for ovarian cancer debulking. The obstruction was due to adhesions that formed a few months after the surgery.
(Courtesy of Cedars-Sinai Medical Center, Los Angeles, CA.)

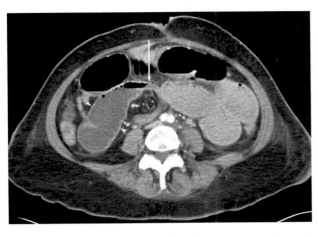

Figure 5-2 • Small-bowel obstruction. CT appearance of a small-bowel obstruction with dilated loops of small bowel filled with gas and fluid. At a transition point *(white arrow),* the bowel narrows and is decompressed distally. This is the point of obstruction and is due to adhesions.
(Courtesy of Cedars-Sinai Medical Center, Los Angeles, CA.)

KEY POINTS

1. Small-bowel obstruction is defined as a mechanical interruption of the normal antegrade transit of intestinal contents.
2. Patients with small bowel obstruction present with abdominal pain, nausea, vomiting, and obstipation.
3. The most common causes are adhesions and hernias.
4. The first test to order is the acute abdominal series.
5. Air-fluid levels and dilated loops of small bowel are the most common radiographic findings.

◼ CROHN DISEASE

Anatomy

Crohn disease is a form of chronic inflammatory bowel disease that classically affects the terminal ileum. It is not limited to this area, however, and may affect any portion of the gastrointestinal GI tract, from the oropharynx to the rectum. Classically it occurs in "skip lesions" where portions of affected bowel are separated by segments of normal bowel. This is in contrast to ulcerative colitis, the other form of inflammatory bowel disease, which affects the colon from the rectum proximally in a continuous fashion.

Etiology

Crohn disease is considered idiopathic. Some pathologists speculate that it is an autoimmune-type disorder that is aggravated by stress, excessive caffeine intake, and smoking cessation. Other theories suggest that it is a chronic infectious process from a yet undiscovered pathogen.

Epidemiology

Incidence is approximately 3 per 100,000 in the United States, and there is some genetic predisposition, with about 15% of patients having a first-degree relative with inflammatory bowel disease. It is more common in whites and affects women more than men in a 1.5-to-1 distribution. The peak age of onset is between 15 and 25, but it may occur later in life.

Pathogenesis

Crohn disease causes deep ulceration of the intestine that involves the mucosa and lamina propria. Aphthous and linear ulcers are seen grossly, and non-caseating granulomas, fissures, and fistulae are seen on microscopic examination of the affected bowel. Crypt abscesses with neutrophils aggregated within mucosal crypt lumens are highly associated with the disease.

Clinical Manifestations

History

Chronic diarrhea that is often blood tinged, fever, abdominal pain, and anorexia are the most common presenting symptoms. Weight loss, fistulae, and intestinal obstruction commonly occur sometime during the course of the disease.

Extraintestinal manifestations, including migratory polyarthritis, sacroiliitis, ankylosing spondylitis, a tendency toward gallstone and renal calculus formation, and erythema nodosum, occur but are not common. There is also an association with sclerosing cholangitis.

Physical Examination

The abdominal examination is less significant than expected. Often patients have only mild abdominal tenderness. Fistulae may be seen on inspection of the perineum. Rectal examination occasionally demonstrates hemepositive stool.

Diagnostic Evaluation

Generally, an upper GI examination with a small-bowel contrast series is the first radiologic test when Crohn disease is suspected. Laboratory evaluation includes elevated erythrocyte sedimentation rate (ESR), hemoglobin level to determine whether anemia is present, and albumin level in severe cases where weight loss has occurred. Colonoscopy with ileoscopy and biopsy can confirm a suspected diagnosis.

Radiologic Findings

On CT scan, thickening of the wall of the terminal ileum raises suspicion for the diagnosis (Figure 5-3). Inflammation of the adjacent mesenteric fat, abscesses, and fistulae often occur in more severe cases. On barium upper GI and small-bowel series examinations, areas of thickened mucosa are seen, classically on the mesenteric side of the bowel. Skip lesions denote areas of affected bowel interspersed between normal-appearing mucosa. Deep, "rose-thorn" ulcerations in the small bowel are often seen (Figure 5-4). Strictures and fistulae to other loops of bowel, bladder, vagina, or skin surface are highly specific for Crohn disease. Generally, plain radiographs are not helpful in the initial diagnosis but may be useful in follow-up if small-bowel obstruction is suspected and in diagnosing extraintestinal manifestations such as sacroiliitis and spondylitis.

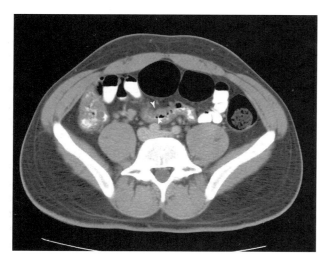

Figure 5-3 • Crohn disease. Patient is a 22-year-old man with inflammation of the terminal ileum consistent with Crohn disease. Oral contrast consisting of dilute Gastrografin is given 1 hour before the scan and helps to distinguish loops of bowel from lymph nodes, vessels, and other abdominal structures.
(Courtesy of Cedars-Sinai Medical Center, Los Angeles, CA.)

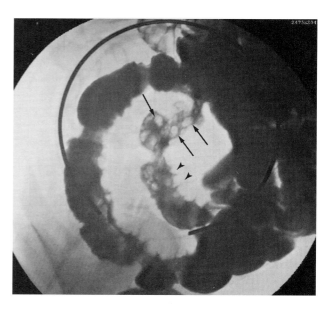

Figure 5-4 • Crohn disease. Spot film from a fluoroscopic small-bowel examination demonstrates a narrowed loop of ileum with a "cobblestone" appearance of the mucosa *(arrows)* and deep "rose thorn" ulcers *(arrowheads)*—findings associated with Crohn disease.
(Courtesy of Cedars-Sinai Medical Center, Los Angeles, CA.)

KEY POINTS

1. Crohn disease is a form of chronic inflammatory bowel disease that classically affects the terminal ileum but may also involve any portion of the GI tract.
2. Chronic diarrhea, fever, abdominal pain, and anorexia are the most common presenting symptoms.
3. On barium examination, areas of thickened mucosa with skip lesions, "rose-thorn" ulcerations, strictures, and fistulae are common findings.

▬ PANCREATITIS

Anatomy

The pancreas is a retroperitoneal structure that is anatomically divided into four portions: the head, including the uncinate process; neck; body; and tail. Its physiologic purpose is to produce and secrete digestive enzymes, insulin, glucagons, and several other enzymes important for digestion and metabolism.

Etiology

Acute pancreatitis occurs as a result of many causes, but it is most commonly associated with ethanol abuse and choledocholithiasis. Other causes include trauma; *Mycoplasma* or Coxsackievirus infection; pancreatic neoplasm; hypercalcemia; hyperlipidemia; and certain medications, including thiazide diuretics, tetracycline, and sulfonamides. Causes of chronic pancreatitis are usually related to alcohol use and biliary tract disease and, less commonly, hyperlipidemia.

Epidemiology

The approximate incidence of pancreatitis is 10 to 20 per 100,000 in the United States. Men and women are generally equally affected. The peak age of incidence is between ages 30 and 40, mostly related to alcohol consumption. There is not usually a genetic association, although there is a rare autosomal-dominant form of inherited predisposition to pancreatitis.

Pathogenesis

The underlying causes are varied, but the mechanism of acute pancreatitis is an inflammatory process that cascades as a result of autodigestion of the gland from the enzymes it produces. Chronic pancreatitis, which is usually associated with chronic alcohol use, results in progressive functional destruction of the gland with exocrine and endocrine deficiencies.

Clinical Manifestations

History

Patients typically present with complaints of mid-epigastric abdominal pain that may radiate through to the back. Nausea, vomiting, and fever are common symptoms. Past medical history may include symptoms of cholelithiasis, including intermittent bouts of postprandial right upper quadrant pain and steatorrhea.

Physical Examination

Fever, jaundice, abdominal tenderness, and absent or diminished bowel sounds are common physical findings. Abdominal distension may occur secondary to a paralytic ileus. More severe cases may have hypotension, tachycardia, and shock physiology. Grey Turner sign with flank discoloration or Cullen sign with umbilical discoloration are also classic physical findings seen in some cases.

Diagnostic Evaluation

Laboratory evaluation includes a serum lipase level in suspected cases. An elevated lipase level is more specific for pancreatitis than a serum amylase level because many other pathologic conditions, such as esophageal rupture, intestinal obstruction, and perforated peptic ulcer, may present with an elevated amylase level and similar symptoms. Ranson criteria, which predict prognosis in pancreatitis, include initial laboratory tests of white blood cell (WBC) count greater than 16,000, serum glucose greater than 200, serum lactate dehydrogenase (LDH) greater than 350, and serum glutamic-oxaloacetic transaminase (SGOT) greater than 250.

Pancreatitis is commonly considered a clinical diagnosis, but imaging is useful, especially in potential surgical cases with pseudocyst or abscess. Radiographic evaluation usually begins with an acute abdominal series, including flat and upright KUB and upright AP chest radiograph. Ultrasound of the abdomen is helpful if the pancreas can be visualized, but it is often obscured by overlying bowel gas. If pancreatitis is high on the differential diagnosis, a CT scan of the abdomen with contrast may confirm the diagnosis. Follow-up CT scans may be performed if there is concern for pseudocyst or abscess formation.

Radiologic Findings

The acute abdominal series often demonstrates a diffuse paralytic ileus pattern. A "sentinel loop" of small bowel in the left upper quadrant represents a focal ileus adjacent to the area of pancreatic inflammation. The "colon cutoff sign" is also strongly associated with pancreatitis and appears as a distended, gas-filled, transverse colon with no colonic gas seen distal to the splenic flexure. A left pleural effusion is a relatively common finding. Calcified gallstones seen on plain radiographs may give an indication as to the cause of pancreatitis.

Ultrasound frequently reveals an edematous, enlarged pancreas, sometimes with dilatation of the pancreatic duct. Gallstones are easily visualized within the gallbladder (GB) on ultrasound; however, the distal body and tail of the pancreas are often poorly visualized by ultrasound, and inflammation in these areas can be missed.

The CT scan can provide a definitive diagnosis of pancreatitis with findings of pancreatic edema, peripancreatic fat inflammation and fluid (Figure 5-5), and pancreatic or common bile duct dilatation (Figure 5-6). IV iodine-based contrast is of value in

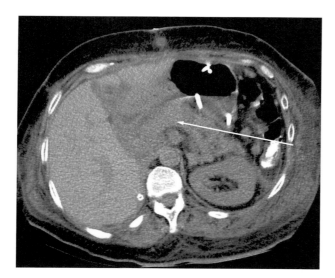

Figure 5-5 • Acute pancreatitis. CT appearance of acute pancreatitis with edema of the pancreas and inflammatory changes *(arrow)* or "stranding" of the peripancreatic fat.
(Courtesy of Cedars-Sinai Medical Center, Los Angeles, CA.)

determining the degree of pancreatic necrosis, which correlates strongly with morbidity. Follow-up CT scans are useful for diagnosing the complications of pancreatitis, such as pseudocyst and abscess formation. Chronic pancreatitis is associated with atrophy

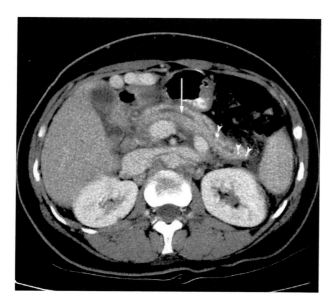

Figure 5-6 • Chronic pancreatitis. Early contrast phase of abdominal CT demonstrating dilated pancreatic duct *(white arrow)*, pancreatic calcifications *(arrowheads)*, and subtle pancreatic inflammation.
(Courtesy of Cedars-Sinai Medical Center, Los Angeles, CA.)

of the gland, scattered calcifications, and pancreatic duct dilatation.

KEY POINTS

1. Acute pancreatitis may occur as a result of many causes, but it is most commonly associated with ethanol intoxication and choledocholithiasis.
2. Patients typically present with complaints of midepigastric abdominal pain that radiates through to the back, nausea, vomiting, and fever.
3. Diagnostic evaluation should include a serum lipase level and an acute abdominal series.
4. A paralytic ileus pattern, "sentinel loop," and "colon cutoff sign" are common radiographic findings associated with pancreatitis.
5. Ultrasound may be useful in some cases if pancreatic edema is demonstrated, but it is often non-specific.
6. CT scan of the abdomen with intravenous contrast frequently provides a definitive diagnosis of pancreatitis with findings of pancreatic edema, peripancreatic fat inflammation and fluid, and pancreatic or common bile duct dilatation.

■ APPENDICITIS

Anatomy

The appendix is a vestigial structure located at the tip of the cecum in the right lower quadrant of the abdomen. Normally it measures less than 5 mm in diameter and has a wall thickness less than 3 mm. It has many anatomic variants in its position and length. It may be closely apposed to the posterior wall of the cecum (retrocecal), adjacent to the right psoas muscle, or in the pelvis.

Etiology

The most common cause of appendicitis is obstruction of the appendiceal lumen, usually by an appendicolith. Other uncommon causes include obstruction by lymphoid tissue hypertrophy or neoplasm, often carcinoid tumor.

Epidemiology

Appendicitis is the most common acute surgical condition, and it will affect about 7% of all people over the course of a lifetime. The incidence is estimated at 10 to 20 per 100,000 in the United States. There is a slight predominance for occurrence of appendicitis in men, especially in adolescents and young adults; however, it can occur at any age.

Pathogenesis

Luminal obstruction leads to bacterial overgrowth and subsequent inflammation. Secondarily there is venous obstruction, ischemia, and necrosis. Some cases progress to appendiceal rupture and peritoneal infection.

Clinical Manifestations

History

Patients present first with anorexia, then with abdominal pain that classically begins in the periumbilical area and then gradually moves to McBurney point, which is located at two thirds the distance from the umbilicus to the right anterior superior iliac spine. Vomiting may occur later as pain increases in the right lower quadrant.

Physical Examination

Rebound tenderness in the right lower quadrant and guarding are classic physical findings of acute appendicitis. Other signs include the psoas sign, which is pain in the deep upper pelvis during extension of a flexed right thigh against examiner resistance. The obturator sign is pain during internal rotation of a flexed right thigh against examiner resistance. A retrocecal appendix may give right flank tenderness to palpation, and an appendix located deep within the pelvis may give local and suprapubic tenderness on rectal examination. Low-grade fever is common at presentation and may increase as symptoms progress. High fevers with peritoneal signs are associated with appendiceal rupture. Often, just after the appendix ruptures, patients notice a sudden decrease in pain.

Diagnostic Evaluation

Appendicitis remains largely a clinical diagnosis. History and physical examination point to the diagnosis, and the laboratory tests and radiographs either confirm or point toward another cause of the symptoms. Laboratory evaluation usually demonstrates an elevated WBC count (10,000 to 20,000) and polymorphonuclear cells (PMNs) greater than 75% on differ-

ential, with a left shift. About 25% of patients will have either hematuria or evidence of WBCs in the urine.

Radiologic evaluation may be very useful in cases of intermediate suspicion based on the history and the physical examination. Generally, plain radiographs are useful as an initial screening study for abdominal pain, but normal findings should not delay the diagnosis when classic findings on the history and physical examination are reported. Both ultrasound (performed preferentially in children and pregnant women) and CT in all other patients are highly accurate studies in diagnosing acute appendicitis. Gastrografin enemas are nonspecific and should not be performed.

Radiologic Findings

On CT scan the appendix is often dilated, greater than 6 mm in transverse diameter. There is often inflammation of the fat surrounding the appendix (Figure 5-7). Adjacent free fluid or a fluid-filled mass may indicate appendiceal perforation. Occasionally a calcified appendicolith is present within the lumen of the appendix and is identified either on a plain abdominal film or on a CT. If rectal contrast has been given, nonfilling of the appendix suggests luminal obstruction and a positive diagnosis (Figure 5-8). If the appendix

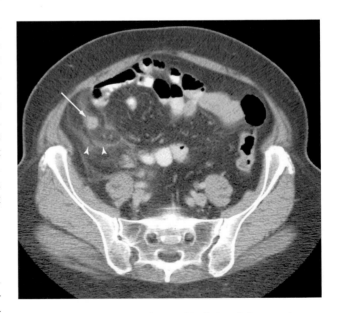

Figure 5-7 • Acute appendicitis. CT of the abdomen demonstrates a dilated, thick-walled appendix seen in cross-section (arrow) with adjacent inflammation of the periappendiceal fat (arrowheads).
(Courtesy of Cedars-Sinai Medical Center, Los Angeles, CA.)

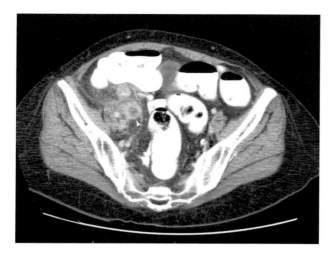

Figure 5-8 • Acute appendicitis. CT with dilute oral contrast demonstrates nonfilling of a markedly dilated appendix and inflammation of the periappendiceal fat.
(Courtesy of Cedars-Sinai Medical Center, Los Angeles, CA.)

completely fills with contrast, then appendicitis is virtually excluded.

Ultrasound examination commonly reveals a dilated, noncompressible tubular structure in the right lower quadrant, representing the appendix (Figure 5-9). This is often seen over the point of maximal tenderness.

Occasionally a calcified appendicolith is seen as a highly echogenic structure with posterior shadowing in the proximal portion of the appendix. Adjacent inflammation and fluid may be seen but are sometimes obscured by overlying bowel gas.

KEY POINTS

1. The most common cause of appendicitis is obstruction of the appendiceal lumen, usually by an appendicolith.
2. Appendicitis is the most common acute surgical condition, and it will affect about 7% of all people over the course of a lifetime.
3. Patients present with anorexia and abdominal pain that begins in the periumbilical area and then moves to McBurney point.
4. Rebound tenderness and guarding in the right lower quadrant are classic physical findings of appendicitis. Other signs include the psoas sign and the obturator sign.
5. Ultrasound examination commonly reveals a dilated, tender, noncompressible tubular structure in the right lower quadrant.
6. On CT scan, stranding of the periappendiceal fat, a dilated appendix greater than 6 mm, and an appendicolith are highly specific findings.

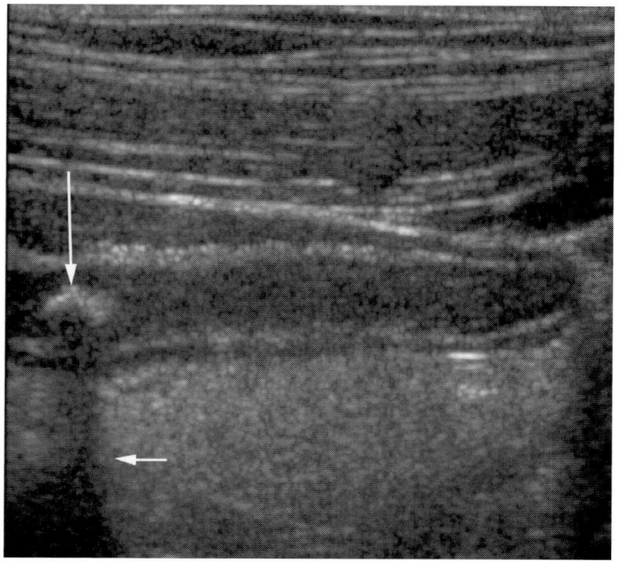

■ DIVERTICULITIS

Anatomy

Colonic diverticula are outpouchings of the mucosa and submucosa through the muscularis layer. They occur at areas of weakness in the muscularis that align along the points where nutrient vessels pierce the muscularis. Diverticula are most commonly located in the sigmoid colon; they are occasionally seen in the ascending, transverse, and descending portions of the colon; and they do not occur in the rectum.

Etiology

The formation of diverticula is thought to occur as a result of a lack of fiber in the diet. High fiber intake allows faster transit through the colon and the formation of softer stool that is easily passed. Slow transit through the colon, hard stool, and higher-than-normal pressures in the sigmoid colon force the mucosa and submucosa out through the weak areas in the muscularis layer, leading to diverticulosis.

Figure 5-9 • Acute appendicitis. Ultrasound of the right lower quadrant demonstrates a noncompressible, thick-walled appendix and an echogenic shadowing *(small arrow)* appendicolith *(large arrow)*.
(Courtesy of Cedars-Sinai Medical Center, Los Angeles, CA.)

Epidemiology

Incidence increases with age and is estimated at 3000 per 100,000 in the United States. It is rare before age 40 and affects men and women equally. There is no genetic predisposition, but it is more common in Western society, likely because of low-fiber diet. Patients with prior history of diverticulitis are at increased risk of developing recurrent episodes.

Pathogenesis

Diverticulitis occurs when diverticula become obstructed and there is subsequent overgrowth of bacteria within the outpouching. The infected diverticulum may have microperforation, causing localized inflammation or frank perforation, leading to abscess formation.

Clinical Manifestations

History

Patients with diverticulosis may be asymptomatic, or they may have intermittent bouts of bleeding. Often diverticula are found incidentally at screening colonoscopy. About 25% of patients with diverticulosis will develop diverticulitis at some point in their life. They often present with left lower quadrant pain, low-grade fever, anorexia, nausea, and vomiting.

Physical Examination

The most common physical findings of diverticulitis are left lower quadrant rebound tenderness, guarding, and palpable mass. Diffuse peritoneal signs such as nonlocalized rebound tenderness or guarding are suggestive of perforation and peritonitis. Bowel sounds may be diminished if paralytic ileus is present.

Diagnostic Evaluation

Radiographs are usually nonspecific, but they may demonstrate evidence of obstruction or ileus (Figure 5-10). CT scan of the abdomen and laboratory evaluation of WBC count are specific for the diagnosis. A CT of the abdomen is useful in determining whether associated abscess formation and safe access for drainage catheter placement are present.

Radiologic Findings

The CT scan frequently demonstrates colonic wall thickening, inflammation of the adjacent mesenteric fat (Figure 5-11), and occasionally small pockets of extraluminal gas suggesting microperforation (Figure 5-12). Diverticula are present in the involved seg-

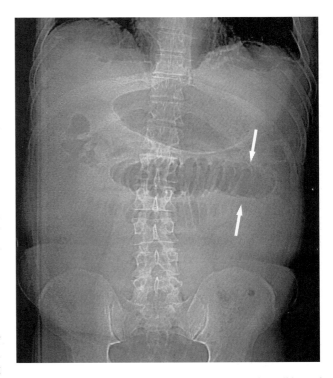

Figure 5-10 • KUB demonstrating dilated loops of small bowel in a pattern of obstruction or ileus. The patient presented with fever, elevated white blood cell count, and left lower quadrant pain and was diagnosed with diverticulitis on CT scan.
(Courtesy of Cedars-Sinai Medical Center, Los Angeles, CA.)

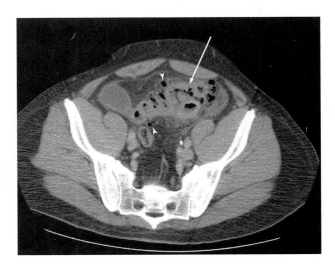

Figure 5-11 • Diverticulitis. CT scan of the same patient in Figure 5-10 demonstrates a thick-walled sigmoid colon with inflammation of the adjacent fat *(white arrow)* and multiple diverticula *(white arrowheads)*.
(Courtesy of Cedars-Sinai Medical Center, Los Angeles, CA.)

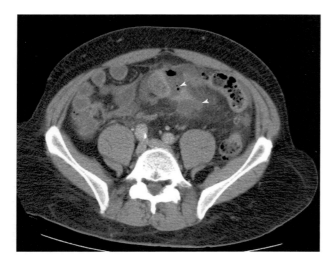

Figure 5-12 • Diverticulitis. CT scan reveals inflammation of the pericolonic fat *(lower arrowhead)* and a small collection of extraluminal gas *(upper arrowhead)* and fluid representing a microperforation from diverticulitis.
(Courtesy of Cedars-Sinai Medical Center, Los Angeles, CA.)

ment of colon. Abscess formation often occurs in the evolution of an episode of diverticulitis. Oral or rectal contrast given before the examination may help in the diagnosis but is not absolutely necessary. A perforated colonic carcinoma may mimic diverticulitis, but more pronounced focal wall thickening or a focal mass is often present.

KEY POINTS

1. Colonic diverticula are outpouchings of the mucosa and submucosa through the muscularis layer, thought to occur because of a lack of fiber in the diet.
2. Diverticulitis occurs when diverticula become obstructed and there is subsequent overgrowth of bacteria.
3. The most common physical findings of diverticulitis are left lower quadrant rebound tenderness, guarding, and palpable mass.
4. CT findings include colonic wall thickening, inflammation of the adjacent mesenteric fat, and small pockets of extraluminal gas and fluid.

■ ACUTE CHOLECYSTITIS

Acute cholecystitis is defined as inflammation of the GB wall, mostly due to cystic duct obstruction.

Anatomy

The GB is located in the GB fossa, through which the plane of separation between the right and left lobes of the liver passes. The GB is covered at least partially by peritoneum—on its posteroinferior surface—which is an explanation for peritoneal signs in cases of GB wall inflammation.

Bile is secreted by the hepatocytes into the bile canaliculi, and then it travels into progressively larger bile ducts. The right and left hepatic ducts merge to form the **common hepatic duct,** which is joined at a right angle by the cystic duct that drains the GB. The newly formed **common bile duct** has a circular muscular sphincter, the choledochal sphincter, located in the region of the duct's entrance into the duodenal wall. This sphincter is distinct from the more distal hepatopancreatic sphincter (of Oddi). When the choledochal sphincter contracts between meals, the bile accumulates along the cystic duct and stores into the GB for concentration and later use (approximately 30 to 60 mL).

Etiology

More than 95% of cases of acute cholecystitis are a consequence of cholelithiasis. A less common disease, acalculous cholecystitis, occurs usually in critically ill patients and in receivers of parenteral nutrition. The etiology of these cases is still not fully understood, but this disease should be thought of in a septic patient where an obvious source is not evident.

Epidemiology

Cholelithiasis (and cholecystitis) occurs in women, in patients with hemolytic anemia, in patients with cirrhosis, and in patients with disease of the distal ileum (i.e., after resection).

Pathogenesis

Formation of most GB calculi is attributed to faulty concentration of bile (cholesterol, bile salts, etc.). If a calculus lodges into the cystic duct during GB contraction, without return into GB during relaxation, obstruction and acute cholecystitis usually occur. Ischemic changes of the GB are thought to be a late change in cases of cholecystitis, not a cause of this disease.

Clinical Manifestations

History

Patients present with postprandial right upper quadrant pain, a symptom of stone engaged into the cystic duct during GB contraction and radiation to the right scapula. Nausea, vomiting, and fever may occur. Some patients present with chest pain mimicking an acute myocardial infarction.

Physical Examination

Leukocytosis, abdominal involuntary guarding, and the Murphy sign (sharp tenderness with stop of inspiration during palpation over the GB) are all indications of the diagnosis.

Most cases of acute cholecystitis are self-limited, lasting less than a week.

Diagnostic Evaluation

Elevated direct bilirubin and alkaline phosphatase are consistent with choledocholithiasis (stones obstructing the common bile duct caudally), a condition more likely to cause complications, particularly if the pancreatic duct becomes obstructed, such as gallstone pancreatitis.

Ultrasound and cholescintigraphy (discussed in Chapter 11) are the modalities of choice for diagnosing acute cholecystitis.

Radiologic Findings

Ultrasound should be used as a confirmatory test when clinical suspicion and laboratory data suggest the diagnosis. In acute cholecystitis, the GB wall is thickened and edematous (it has an echolucent line through it), and the GB may contain stones (Figure 5-13). In gan-

grenous cholecystitis, the GB wall is asymmetrically thickened, and multiple echolucent layers are present. The positive sonographic Murphy sign refers to eliciting maximum tenderness by pressing the ultrasound transducer over the GB.

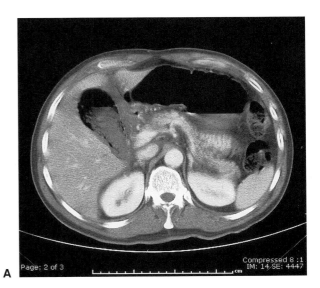

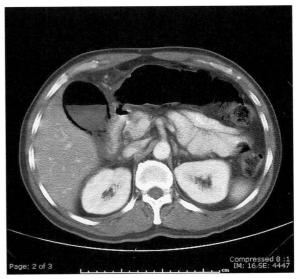

Figure 5-14 • A: Acute cholecystitis. Although not an indicated modality for this diagnosis, this CT scan demonstrates a case of acute emphysematous cholecystitis. Gas is outlining the gallbladder (GB) wall and is also present within the lumen (horizontal gas-fluid level). The common bile duct (CBD) is normal in caliber. **B:** Acute cholecystitis. Lower axial image demonstrates "fat stranding" around the GB.
(Courtesy of University of Southern California Medical Center, Los Angeles, CA.)

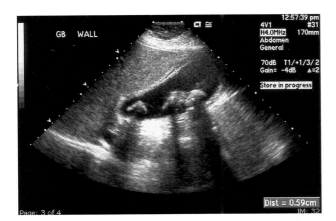

Figure 5-13 • Acute cholecystitis. Ultrasound shows a thickened gallbladder wall (normal measurement is <3 mm) and a small volume of pericholecystic fluid.
(Courtesy of University of Southern California Medical Center, Los Angeles, CA.)

CT should be used only in complicated cases of cholecystitis for obtaining additional information (i.e., associated pancreatitis, cholecystoenteric fistula formation, abscess development). The findings on CT, although not the study of choice, are demonstrated in Figure 5-14.

Magnetic resonance cholangiopancreatography (MRCP) has a role in imaging stones within the common bile duct (choledocholithiasis), when this structure cannot be well imaged by sonography (due to overlying gas, or in obese patients), and when contraindications to endoscopic retrograde cholangiopancreatography exist. MRCP is a noninvasive modality through which three-dimensional reconstructions of the biliary tree are obtained.

KEY POINTS

1. Acute cholecystitis is not always secondary to gallstones. Diabetes mellitus, prolonged parenteral nutrition, and other severe illnesses can cause cholecystitis (acalculous cholecystitis constitutes 5% to 10% of cholecystitis cases).
2. Ultrasound and hepatobiliary nuclear medicine scans are the optimal diagnostic imaging modalities.
3. CT is a poor tool for diagnosing uncomplicated acute cholecystitis, but it should be used in evaluating the pancreas in gallstone pancreatitis or if other complications are suspected (abscess or fistula).

Urologic Imaging

■ NEPHROLITHIASIS

Anatomy

Renal calculi occur throughout the urinary tract and may be seen incidentally on plain films overlying the renal shadow, in the ureter, or in the bladder. They initially form in the proximal urinary tract and may move distally, sometimes passing during urination. The three most common points where they become obstructed are the ureteropelvic junction (UPJ), the point where the ureter crosses over the iliac vessels, and the ureterovesicular junction (UVJ) (Figure 6-1).

Etiology

Renal stones are generally of four basic types (Box 6-1). A small percentage (<1%) of stones also occur as

BOX 6-1	FOUR BASIC TYPES OF RENAL STONES

1. Calcium oxalate or calcium phosphate (75%)
2. Struvite (magnesium ammonium phosphate) (about 15%) associated with alkalinized urine and infections
3. Uric acid (8%) associated with gout and multiple myeloma
4. Cystine (2%) stones associated with cystinuria

precipitates of medications. One of these medications is indinavir, a common human immunodeficiency virus (HIV) protease inhibitor. The stones from indinavir are notable because, unlike the other types of stones, they are nonopaque and are not visible on a noncontrast CT.

Epidemiology

Patients usually present between the ages of 30 and 50. Predisposing conditions include Crohn disease, calyceal diverticula, hypercalcemia, and renal tubular acidosis. Calcium stones are more common in men at a 3:1 ratio with women. Struvite stones are slightly more common in women. About 1 in 10 people will have renal stones at some point during their lifetime.

Pathogenesis

Stones form when urine becomes supersaturated with crystals, which begin to precipitate. Precipitation may be increased or decreased, depending on the pH of the urine and the type of crystal being formed.

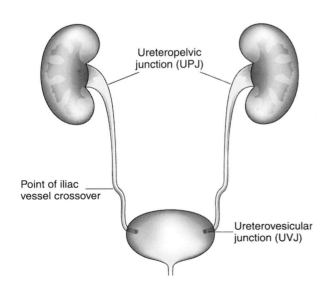

Figure 6-1 • Common points of ureteral obstruction from calculi.

Clinical Manifestations

History

Patients with nephrolithiasis often present with flank pain known as "renal colic" that waxes and wanes as the ureter contracts against the stone. The pain may radiate to the bladder area or groin.

Physical Examination

On examination, there is pain at the costovertebral angle on the affected side. Some patients have chills and fever if there is an associated infection. Hematuria is common; however, it may be microscopic rather than gross.

Diagnostic Evaluation

An elevated WBC with predominant granulocytes is common on laboratory evaluation. Plain films of the abdomen demonstrate a calcification in 80% to 90% of patients, but small stones in the pelvis are difficult to distinguish from phleboliths. Urate calculi are radiolucent on plain radiographs. Historically the intravenous pyelogram (IVP) was the diagnostic test of choice to evaluate for obstruction and to determine the size and location of calculi. The CT urogram without contrast has replaced the IVP. It is performed much faster, avoids the risks of iodinated contrast, and has a decreased radiation dose to the patient compared with an IVP. A decreased radiation dose is especially important to patients of child-bearing age, because a significant amount of radiation is delivered to the pelvis and gonads during an IVP. Ultrasound of the kidneys also shows calcifications as echo densities with posterior shadowing. Hydronephrosis is commonly visualized with ultrasound if there is an obstructing stone; however, ultrasound is inherently neither as sensitive nor as specific as CT in diagnosing ureteral obstruction.

Radiologic Findings

Historically the first imaging study performed for suspected nephrolithiasis has been the KUB to evaluate for calcifications. About 80% to 90% of urinary tract calculi will appear radiodense on plain radiographs. Urate crystals are not well visualized on plain radiographs. Some clinicians order an IVP to confirm a suspected calcification seen on plain radiographs. Contrast material concentrates in the kidneys and provides information about the size of the kidneys and their relative function. The affected kidney may appear larger with a persistent nephrogram. There is delayed opacification of the collecting system on the affected side. A urinary tract calculus appears as a filling defect in the collecting system or ureter. Hydronephrosis or hydroureter may be present, depending on the level of obstruction.

The noncontrast CT urogram has replaced the KUB and IVP as the preferred method of imaging in suspected nephrolithiasis. The risks of contrast are avoided, the radiation dose is reduced, and in most cases the examination can be performed and interpreted in much less time. Nearly all renal calculi will appear as high attenuation on CT, with the exception of indinavir precipitates. The main finding in acute urolithiasis on CT is a calcification in the affected collecting system (Figure 6-2 A, B), ureter, or bladder. Mild hydronephrosis often persists after the stone has already passed. Other findings that may support the diagnosis include inflammation and fluid in the perinephric fat caused by edema or urine released from a ruptured fornix. Stones in the ureter that are larger than 7 mm rarely pass, but smaller stones in the distal ureter commonly pass with time.

KEY POINTS

1. The noncontrast CT urogram has replaced the IVP in most imaging centers as the modality of choice in the evaluation of suspected urolithiasis.
2. The diagnosis of urolithiasis is made with CT when an obstructing stone is visualized and associated with dilatation of the proximal ureter or collecting system.
3. Calcifications are seen at the UPJ, the point where the ureter crosses over the iliac vessels, and at the UVJ.

▨ TESTICULAR TORSION

Anatomy

The testes are suspended within the scrotum by the spermatic cords. The spermatic cords contain the ductus deferens and the blood vessels, nerves, and lymphatics for the testes. The testes are covered by the dense, fibrous tunica albuginea, which is partially covered by the visceral and parietal layers of the tunica vaginalis. The testes are normally fixed in place within the scrotum by the gubernaculum.

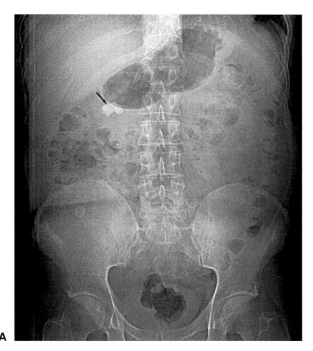

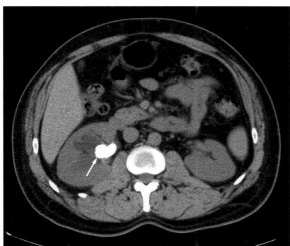

Figure 6-2 • A: Urolithiasis. KUB demonstrates a large right renal calcification. **B:** Urolithiasis. CT of the same patient in (A) with right renal collecting system calculus.
(Courtesy of Cedars-Sinai Medical Center, Los Angeles, CA.)

Etiology

Testicular torsion is a true radiographic emergency. It is caused by rotation of the testis and spermatic cord, causing venous and eventually arterial occlusion and subsequent infarction of the affected testis. Trauma or strenuous physical exertion is often the cause.

Epidemiology

Torsion presents at any age, but it most commonly occurs in two peaks: in neonates and in the second decade of life.

Pathogenesis

The bell-clapper deformity is a congenital anatomic variant in which there is congenital absence of the **gubernaculum,** the posterior attachment of the tunica vaginalis to the scrotum. With a bell-clapper deformity, the testis is only loosely connected to the scrotum and is able to move freely within the scrotal sac and twist **(torse)** around the axis of the blood vessels (Figure 6-3). The bell-clapper variant is bilateral in 50% to 80% of cases.

Clinical Manifestations

History

Patients usually present with sudden onset of testicular pain, which increases in severity as ischemia progresses.

Physical Examination

On examination, the affected testis is tender, enlarged, and may be edematous and erythematous.

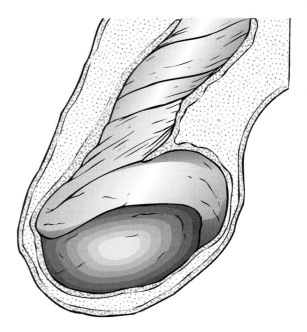

Figure 6-3 • Testicular torsion due to bell-clapper deformity.
(Used with permission from Karp SJ, Morris JPG, Soybel DI. *Blueprints Surgery,* 3rd ed. Malden, MA: Blackwell Publishing, 2004.)

It is often located high in the scrotum, sometimes oriented with the long axis horizontal rather than in the normal vertical position. There may be an absent cremasteric reflex, which is the normal retraction of the scrotum and testis when the ipsilateral inner thigh is lightly scratched. The presentation often mimics epididymo-orchitis and an incarcerated inguinal hernia, the two major differential diagnostic considerations. Other differential diagnoses include traumatic hematoma, varicocele, hydrocele, scrotal abscess, and testicular tumor.

Diagnostic Evaluation

Ultrasonography with Doppler and nuclear scintigraphy are two commonly used imaging modalities; however, ultrasound can be performed more rapidly and is the test of choice. Other diagnoses that may mimic torsion, such as epididymitis and orchitis, can be diagnosed with ultrasound as well. Rapid diagnosis and treatment of testicular torsion are essential because the salvage rate drops off quickly after 6 hours. At 12 hours, the salvage rate is about 20%. At 24 hours the chance of salvage is virtually zero.

Radiologic Findings

Ultrasound with color-flow Doppler reveals absent or decreased blood flow (Figure 6-4A, B) in the affected testis during the acute period (<6 hours). Comparison is made to the unaffected side. During the acute period, testicular torsion can be distinguished from epididymo-orchitis, which has increased blood flow as a result of the inflammatory process. Incarcerated inguinal hernia will have normal blood flow to the testis, and ultrasound may reveal the contents of the

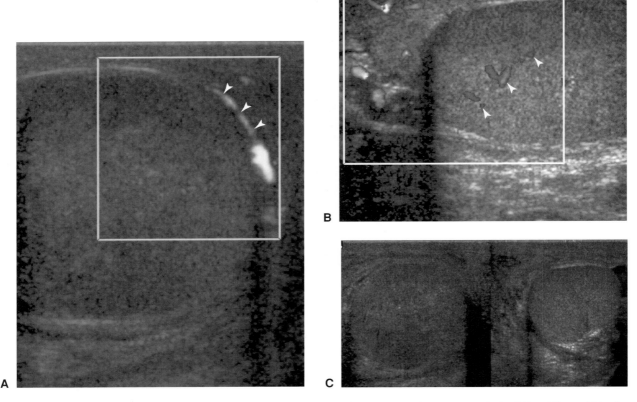

Figure 6-4 • A: Testicular torsion. Ultrasound of the testis with Doppler flow imaging demonstrates lack of blood flow within the torsed right testis. There is flow peripherally. **B:** Normal Doppler flow ultrasound in left testis of the same patient as in (A). *Arrowheads* show areas of blood flow. **C:** Testicular torsion. Side-by-side comparison with gray-scale ultrasound reveals heterogeneous echotexture of the torsed right testis compared with the normal left testis. The patient had the acute onset of pain after falling from a skateboard.
(Courtesy of Cedars-Sinai Medical Center, Los Angeles, CA.)

hernia. During the late period (>24 hours), gray scale ultrasound imaging shows heterogeneity of the affected testis (Figure 6-4C) and absent blood flow within the testis itself. Blood flow may increase blood flow with color-flow Doppler around the periphery of the testis as inflammation increases.

Nuclear scintigraphy may be used as an adjunct to testicular ultrasound imaging. It is not used in children younger than 2 years old because the testes are too small to be identified by the gamma cameras. The finding of a unilateral "cold" or photopenic testis is positive for testicular torsion. Another sign used to identify testicular torsion on nuclear imaging is the "ring sign." With this finding, activity around the testis with a central photopenic zone of no activity signifies inflammation around an ischemic or necrotic testis.

KEY POINTS

1. Testicular torsion is a true radiographic emergency. It is caused by rotation of the testis and spermatic cord, causing venous and eventually arterial occlusion and subsequent infarction of the affected testis.
2. The bell-clapper deformity is a risk factor.
3. The two major differential diagnostic considerations are epididymo-orchitis and an incarcerated inguinal hernia.
4. Ultrasound with Doppler color-flow imaging is the test of choice, and it reveals absent or decreased blood flow in the affected testis during the acute period (<6 hours).

◼ URINARY TRACT NEOPLASMS

Anatomy

Urinary tract neoplasms involve either the renal parenchyma or the collecting system (from renal calyces to the urethra). The most common malignant neoplasm of the kidney is renal cell carcinoma (80% to 90% of the renal malignancies). The principal site of occurrence of cancer within the collecting system is the urinary bladder.

Etiology

Transitional cell carcinoma is attributed to exposure to aniline dyes, postradiation treatment of other tumors of the pelvis, recurrent or chronic cystitis, and smoking. The relatively uncommon squamous cell carcinoma of the urinary bladder is frequently associated with bladder calculi and chronic infection (a frequently mentioned infectious agent endemic in third world countries is the parasite *Schistosoma haematobium*).

Epidemiology

Urinary tract malignancies are thought to be more frequent in smokers, and males are more affected than females.

Clinical Manifestations

History

Painless hematuria is the most common complaint in urinary tract tumors.

Physical Examination

Some patients are discovered to have microscopic hematuria at a routine physical examination, whereas others present with flank pain and a mass. Occasionally a renal cell carcinoma may be incidentally discovered on a CT or ultrasound ordered for other reasons.

Diagnostic Evaluation

An important imaging assessment in renal cell carcinoma is the evaluation for venous involvement (spread into the renal veins and into inferior vena cava) for surgical planning. Ultrasound with color flow, MRI, or CT can determine venous tumor spread. Renal cell carcinoma is diagnosed by imaging, and, if a tumor is resectable, surgical excision should be performed without preliminary biopsy (biopsy is thought to spread a potentially curable neoplasm).

In urinary tract malignant neoplasms, attention should be directed to detection of any additional synchronous tumors, particularly for transitional cell carcinoma, because tumor of the ureter can spread to the urinary bladder.

CT and MRI are reliable tools for the evaluation of invasion of urothelial tumor into adjacent structures and for metastases, but both give limited information regarding the local tumor (i.e., they cannot appreciate the depth of invasion into the urinary bladder layers).

Radiologic Findings

Enhancing lesions within the renal parenchyma or in the collecting system are likely carcinomas (Figure 6-5A).

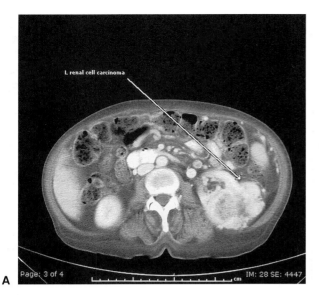

L renal cell carcinoma

A Page: 3 of 4   IM: 28 SE: 4447

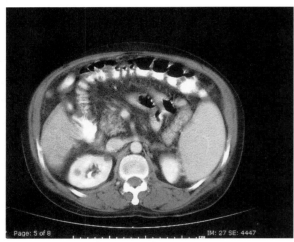

B Page: 5 of 8   IM: 27 SE: 4447

Figure 6-5 • A: Renal cell carcinoma (hypernephroma). Contrast-enhanced CT demonstrates a mass in the left kidney, proven at surgery to be adenocarcinoma of the kidney. **B:** Renal cysts demonstrate a density lower than the renal parenchyma and do not enhance postcontrast administration.
(Courtesy of University of Southern California Medical Center, Los Angeles, CA.)

Enhancement is determined by comparing images before and after the administration of intravenous contrast. A nonenhancing spherical structure within the kidney with density near that of water is more likely to represent a renal cyst (Figure 6-5B). At times a renal ultrasound is recommended for elucidation because it is a good modality for distinguishing cystic from solid lesions. Simple cysts are a common occurrence, but complex cysts (with septations or solid components) need to be followed up or treated as potential carcinomas.

Ultrasound is a good modality for distinguishing a bland versus a tumor thrombus invading the renal veins or the IVC. The tumor thrombus demonstrates color flow within, representing its vascular supply.

Circumferential urinary bladder wall thickening may be due to involvement by tumor, or may be secondary to cystitis or hypertrophy resulting from obstructive physiology. An area of eccentric bladder wall enhancement is most likely a carcinoma (Figure 6-6). The definitive diagnosis is obtained by cystoscopy with biopsy, especially since many urinary bladder cancers may not be identified by imaging.

KEY POINTS

1. CT with intravenous contrast or MRI can be ordered for urinary tract malignancies for staging.
2. Ultrasound is appropriate to determine venous invasion in renal cell carcinoma.
3. A negative imaging study does not exclude the presence of a urothelial neoplasm.

■ PROSTATE CARCINOMA

Etiology

Carcinoma of the prostate is attributed to hormonal influences on the androgen-sensitive neoplastic cells.

Epidemiology

Prostate carcinoma is the second most common cause of cancer death in men in the United States, and it constitutes about 20% of all cancers. Prostate carcinoma is generally a disease of males over the age of 50.

Pathogenesis

The periphery of the gland is the most common site of origin of prostate carcinoma (70%). This tumor spreads to contiguous tissues as well as to remote sites through veins and lymphatics.

Clinical Manifestations

History

Most patients have no symptoms or present with low back pain resulting from metastatic osseous involvement.

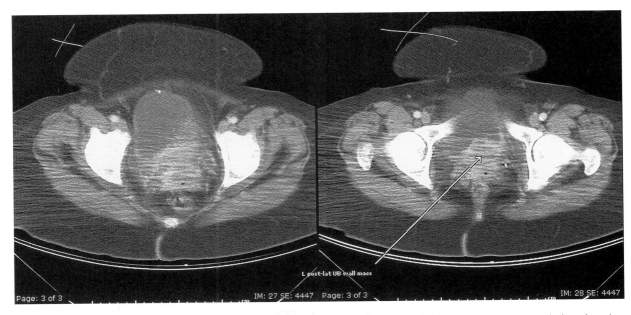

Figure 6-6 • Transitional cell carcinoma of the urinary bladder. Contrast-enhanced CT demonstrates an irregularly enhancing area in the left posterolateral urinary bladder wall, forming a mass. Image on the left shows a larger portion of the urine-filled urinary bladder.
(Courtesy of University of Southern California Medical Center, Los Angeles, CA.)

Physical Examination

On rectal examination, an indurated gland or nodules are found.

Diagnostic Evaluation

Prostate-specific antigen (PSA), although not prostate cancer specific, is currently widely used in conjunction with a digital rectal examination for cancer screening of men over the age of 50. This test is considered to be most helpful as a marker in cancer follow-up because mildly elevated levels can be seen in noncancerous conditions (e.g., in benign prostatic hyperplasia). The digital examination discovers a hardened gland resulting from infiltration with tumor.

Once advanced prostate carcinoma is diagnosed, a bone scintigraphy is indicated to evaluate for bone metastases. If radiculopathy or cord compression is suspected, an MRI of the appropriate level of the spine is warranted to evaluate for possible extension of tumor into spinal canal. CT (Figure 6-7) is used to assess the degree of involvement of the pelvic sidewalls, urinary bladder, seminal vesicles, and lymph nodes, and it is used for staging. Ultrasound is used for biopsy guidance.

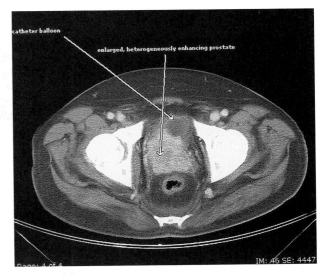

Figure 6-7 • Prostate carcinoma. Iodinated contrast-enhanced CT demonstrates a large prostate gland with irregular borders and heterogeneous enhancement.
(Courtesy of University of Southern California Medical Center, Los Angeles, CA.)

Radiologic Findings

The bone scan is a valuable modality for detection of bone metastases (blastic lesions demonstrate good uptake on the bone scan).

Asymmetric enlargement of the seminal vesicles signals involvement of these glands with tumor. Absence of a fat plane between the prostate and the urinary bladder likely represents tumor spread. Lymph-node carcinomatous involvement may not always be easily appreciated because some of the affected lymph nodes are not enlarged, and very subtle changes (enhancement and mild adjacent fat stranding) are the only clue.

KEY POINTS

1. CT with intravenous contrast or MRI is usually obtained to stage prostate carcinoma.
2. Bone scan is the study of choice to evaluate for osseous metastases.
3. Transrectal prostate biopsy is performed with ultrasound guidance.
4. If spinal cord involvement is suspected, obtain an MRI to evaluate the extent of cord compression.

GENERAL ANATOMY

The adnexal structures, including the ovaries, fallopian tubes, and ovarian vessels, are connected to the uterus by the broad ligament. The fimbriae of the fallopian tubes wrap around the ovaries but are also open to the peritoneal cavity. An ovum released from an ovarian follicle remains free in the peritoneal cavity for a brief time before being swept into the fallopian tube by the fimbriae (Figure 7-1).

ECTOPIC PREGNANCY

Anatomy

Ectopic pregnancy results when implantation occurs outside the uterine cavity. By far the most common site is the fallopian tube, but other possible locations include the ovary, the abdomen, or the endocervix.

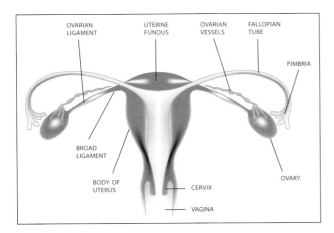

Figure 7-1 • Normal anatomy of the female reproductive organs.

Etiology

A heterotopic pregnancy is a rare twin gestation when one embryo implants within the endometrial cavity and the other one outside.

Epidemiology

Ectopic pregnancy can occur at any reproductive age. Rates of ectopic pregnancy have increased over the years, and a higher prevalence of sexually transmitted diseases (STDs) has been postulated as a cause.

Pathogenesis

Ectopic pregnancy is usually the result of previously damaged fallopian tubes. When normal fertilization occurs in the distal portion of the tube, the conceptus traverses the proximal tube to implant within the uterine cavity. Any structural or functional distortion of the fallopian tube prevents this normal process. One of the most common reasons is infection from STDs, such as *Neisseria gonorrheae* and *Chlamydia trachomatis*. Prior abdominal surgery can cause adhesive disease, leading to partial obstruction or to structurally altered uterine tubes.

Clinical Manifestations

History

The most common complaint is intermittent or constant lower abdominal pain and, less commonly, bleeding. Many women are not aware of being pregnant at the time of presentation.

Physical Examination

Abdominal tenderness with palpation is usually localized to the right or left lower quadrants, but some patients have diffuse pain. Bimanual examination may help to localize this sign further, but care should be excercised to avoid iatrogenic rupture of the ectopic pregnancy. Inability to elicit pain does not exclude an ectopic pregnancy.

Diagnostic Evaluation

The combination of quantitative serum beta human chorionic gonadotropin hormone (beta-hCG) values and transvaginal ultrasound are the standard for diagnosis. The principles involved in making the diagnosis rely on the levels of beta-hCG being well correlated with a certain gestational age. At a beta-HCG level of 1500 mIU per milliliter, called the **discriminatory zone,** a normal intrauterine pregnancy should be visualized by ultrasound. Absence of an intrauterine pregnancy meets the criterion for the label of abnormal pregnancy.

Radiologic Findings

Many times an extrauterine mass can be visualized by ultrasound, further supporting the clinical diagnosis. The usual finding is a mass located between the uterus and ovary (Figure 7-2), but if no mass can be identified transvaginally, a transabdominal ultrasound (a probe placed on the abdominal wall using a fully distended urinary bladder as a window for imaging) should also be performed. The mass has the characteristics of an early gestation with an echolucent

(dark) center surrounded by echogenic tissue. If the ectopic pregnancy is advanced, a fetal pole and even cardiac motion can be detected. Sometimes the outline of the fallopian tube can be appreciated sonographically.

Evaluation of the uterus may be normal, but a pseudogestational sac (blood in the endometrial cavity) can sometimes be identified. If the conceptus implants within one of the cornua of the uterus (the portion of the uterus where the tube enters), a complete ring of myometrium is seen around the gestational sac. A large volume of free fluid in the cul-de-sac is due to hemoperitoneum resulting from rupture of the tube.

KEY POINTS

1. Ectopic pregnancy is a challenging clinical diagnosis, and the increase in number of cases is attributed to a rise in STDs.
2. Ultrasound is the imaging study of choice for aiding in diagnosing an ectopic pregnancy.
3. A normal transvaginal ultrasound does not exclude an ectopic pregnancy. Efforts should be made to locate the ectopic pregnancy by transabdominal ultrasound.
4. A complex (echogenic and echolucent component) adnexal mass, the absence of a normal intrauterine pregnancy, and correlation with a positive beta-hCG is 95% diagnostic.
5. Visualization of cardiac activity in the extrauterine mass is diagnostic.

■ OVARIAN TORSION

Etiology

Ovarian torsion is a result of rotation of the ovary around its vascular supply. Adnexal mass is usually the cause because the ovarian ligament and the broad ligament cannot support the weight of the mass in the normal anatomic position. Common adnexal masses include ovarian neoplasms, polycystic ovary, large ovarian cysts, endometriomas, and dermoid cysts (Figure 7-3).

Epidemiology

Ovarian torsion occurs in women of any age, but it is most common in childhood and adolescence. In

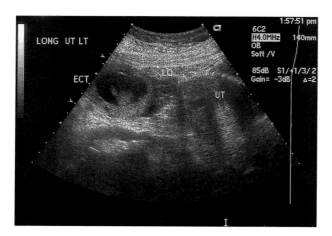

Figure 7-2 • Ectopic pregnancy. Ultrasound demonstrates a left adnexal ectopic pregnancy (ECT) adjacent to the left ovary (LO). The uterus (UT) contained no gestational sac.
(Courtesy of University of Southern California Medical Center, Los Angeles, CA.)

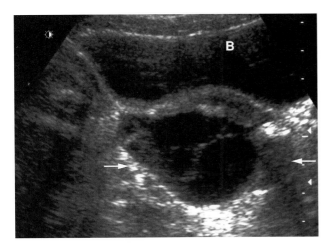

Figure 7-3 • Dermoid cyst. Ultrasound of the pelvis demonstrates a complex cystic mass in the adnexa, which was found to be a dermoid cyst.
(Courtesy of Cedars-Sinai Medical Center, Los Angeles, CA.)

childhood the cause is usually a large dermoid tumor (teratoma), which is the most common ovarian tumor in preadolescent women. In young adult women, large ovarian cysts are the most common cause of torsion. In postmenopausal women, ovarian adenocarcinoma is the most common cause.

Pathogenesis

When ovarian torsion occurs, venous return is obstructed and the ovary becomes edematous. The edema adds to the weight and volume of the ovary, often leading to further torsion. The ovary becomes ischemic because of the reduced flow of arterial blood, especially in small and medium-sized vessels.

Clinical Manifestations

History

Women often present to the emergency department complaining of extreme acute-onset pelvic pain. The acute nature of the pain relates to the fact that a slow-growing mass may not cause pain, but when it acts as a lead point for torsion, the subsequent ischemia to the affected ovary is acutely painful.

Physical Examination

With ovarian torsion, there is often deep pain to palpation on the affected side of the pelvis and often generalized pelvic pain. On physical examination, ovarian torsion may mimic appendicitis, with right lower quadrant tenderness, or diverticulitis, with left lower quadrant tenderness. Palpation for adnexal masses during the pelvic examination is important because these masses are frequently an underlying cause of ovarian torsion. Vaginal bleeding is not commonly associated with torsion.

Diagnostic Evaluation

Ultrasound is the imaging study of choice in evaluating acute pelvic pain or suspected pelvic mass. The test can be performed quickly and easily from the emergency department without the need for preparation. Transvaginal ultrasound provides detailed anatomy of the uterus and adnexae. If ovarian torsion is suspected, the diagnosis should be made within 4 hours to save the ovary from infarction. Doppler imaging should be a part of the examination to evaluate the blood flow to the affected ovary. Alternatively, MRI of the pelvis without contrast can be done, but it may take up to 1 hour to perform, and there must be no contraindications to MRI, such as the presence of a pacemaker, intracranial aneurysm clips, or intraorbital metallic foreign bodies.

Laboratory tests should be performed to exclude pregnancy as a cause of the pelvic pain. Other tests, including complete blood count (CBC) and WBC count, are usually normal with ovarian torsion. This may help in excluding pelvic inflammatory disease, tubo-ovarian abscess, or other infectious and inflammatory causes of pelvic pain from the differential diagnosis (Box 7-1).

Radiologic Findings

An adnexal mass greater than 2.5 cm on the side of the pain is the most common ultrasonographic finding

BOX 7-1	DIFFERENTIAL DIAGNOSIS OF ACUTE PELVIC PAIN

- Ruptured ovarian follicle (most common)
- Endometriosis
- Pelvic inflammatory disease
- Tubo-ovarian abscess
- Ectopic pregnancy
- Ovarian torsion
- Nongynecologic causes
  - Appendicitis
  - Diverticulitis

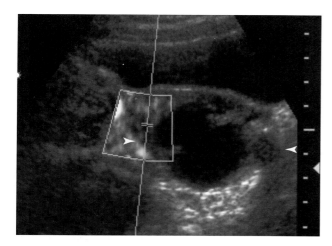

Figure 7-4 • Ovarian mass. Ultrasound image of complex cystic and solid ovarian mass. The cursor is placed over an area of blood flow to evaluate for potential torsion.
(Courtesy of Cedars-Sinai Medical Center, Los Angeles, CA.)

in ovarian torsion (Figure 7-4). This nonspecific finding becomes important only when the history, physical examination, and other findings direct the differential diagnosis toward ovarian torsion. Absence or severe reduction of venous blood flow to the ovary on Doppler color flow imaging (Figure 7-5) is a useful finding, although it is not diagnostic. However, if venous flow is noted centrally within the ovary, torsion is virtually excluded.

A unilateral enlarged ovary with multiple peripheral cortical follicles and pelvic free fluid are also common nonspecific findings. The free fluid commonly seen with torsion represents hemorrhage from a necrotic ovary following prolonged arterial occlusion and subsequent ischemia.

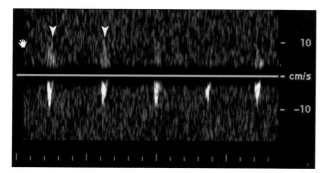

Figure 7-5 • Ovarian torsion. Doppler flow tracing demonstrates only arterial blood flow. No venous flow could be identified in the ovary shown in Figure 7-3.
(Courtesy of Cedars-Sinai Medical Center, Los Angeles, CA.)

KEY POINTS

1. Ovarian torsion is a result of rotation of the ovary around its vascular supply.
2. The most common presenting complaint is acute-onset, extreme pelvic pain.
3. Ultrasound is the imaging study of choice.
4. The diagnosis of ovarian torsion should be made quickly (<4 hours) to save the ovary from infarction.
5. A nonspecific ovarian mass on the side of the pain is the most common ultrasonographic finding in ovarian torsion.
6. Absence of severe reduction of venous blood flow to the ovary on Doppler color-flow imaging is a useful finding, although it is not diagnostic.
7. Venous blood flow centrally within the ovary virtually excludes ovarian torsion.

◼ OVARIAN CARCINOMA

Etiology

Primary ovarian neoplasms are grouped according to the cell type of origin. The ovary is composed of germ cells, stromal or supporting cells, and epithelial cells, all of which may give rise to a neoplasm. Epithelial cells that cover the surface of the ovaries give rise to serous or mucinous cystadenocarcinomas, clear cell carcinomas, and endometrioid carcinomas. Germ cells or oocytes are the cells of origin for dysgerminomas, embryonal cell cancers, choriocarcinomas, yolk sac tumors, and teratomas (dermoids). Stromal cells give rise to granulosa cell tumors, Sertoli-Leydig cell tumors, and fibromas. Other tumors of the ovaries include lymphoma and metastatic tumors commonly from breast, uterine, or GI primary malignancies (known as **Krukenberg tumors** when they metastasize to the ovary).

Epidemiology

Ovarian carcinoma is the fifth leading cause of cancer death in women, and it constitutes 25% of all gynecologic malignancies. The incidence is approximately 20,000 new cases each year, with peak incidence at ages 50 to 60. Epithelial cell neoplasms (75% of ovarian tumors) occur in the fifth to eighth decades. Germ cell tumors (15%) occur more often in women aged 12 to 40, although epithelial cell neoplasm is the most common neoplasm in this age group. Stromal tumors make up the remaining 5% to 10% of ovarian tumors.

There is some genetic component to ovarian cancer, with an increased relative risk of 1.5 if two first-degree relatives have had the disease. The *BRCA-1* gene has been implicated in many cases with such genetic predisposition.

Clinical Manifestations

History

Patients often consult their primary care physician with nonspecific complaints of weight loss, abdominal distension, vague abdominal and pelvic discomfort, or the feeling of a pelvic mass. Some patients may present acutely if the mass is large enough to cause torsion and acute pelvic pain. Risk factors that should be elicited during the medical history are low parity, high-fat high-lactose diet, and delayed childbearing. Oral contraceptive pills statistically have a protective effect.

Physical Examination

Ascites, pelvic mass, and cachexia are late signs found on physical examination. Unfortunately ovarian neoplasms often present at an advanced stage, often with distant metastases, with 65% of patients having metastatic disease at diagnosis. Although cancer antigen 125 (CA-125) levels are elevated in most patients with the disease, the test is not specific for ovarian neoplasm and is generally not used as a screening tool; rather, it is used as a way to follow treatment effectiveness in confirmed cases.

Diagnostic Evaluation

Pelvic ultrasound is the imaging modality most often used for suspected ovarian neoplasm. Both transabdominal and transvaginal imaging should be performed. The transabdominal views provide a general survey of the pelvis to evaluate the upper pelvic structures, to look for lymphadenopathy or peritoneal spread, and to find pelvic free fluid. Transvaginal images define with greater detail the extent of disease in the ovary and adnexa. If torsion is suspected, Doppler imaging should also be performed. The differential diagnosis of an ovarian mass includes both benign and malignant neoplasms, ovarian cysts, torsion, and endometrioma.

Radiologic Findings

The most common ultrasonographic finding with ovarian carcinoma is a unilateral adnexal mass with

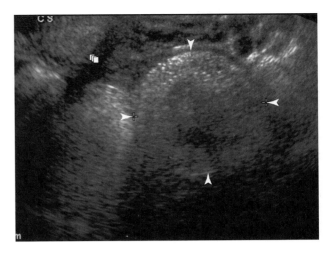

Figure 7-6 • Ovarian carcinoma. Ultrasound of large, heterogeneous, echogenic adnexal mass.
(Courtesy of Cedars-Sinai Medical Center, Los Angeles, CA.)

complex cystic features (Figure 7-6). If the volume of the ovary is greater than 18 cm³ in premenopausal women or greater than 8 cm³ in postmenopausal women, it is considered abnormal and suspicious for ovarian neoplasm. Mixed cystic and solid lesions are suggestive of malignancy and occur most commonly with ovarian cystadenocarcinomas (Figure 7-7). Cystic components are identified by a lack of internal echoes (i.e., they appear black on ultrasound) and posterior acoustic enhancement (brightness beyond the cyst). A cyst larger than 3.5 cm (larger than the usual maturating follicles) should be followed with ultrasound for resolution.

Other findings that suggest malignancy are listed in Box 7-2.

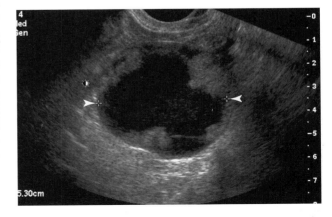

Figure 7-7 • Ovarian cystadenocarcinoma. Ultrasound images of mixed cystic and solid ovarian mass.
(Courtesy of Cedars-Sinai Medical Center, Los Angeles, CA.)

BOX 7-2	ULTRASONOGRAPHIC FINDINGS THAT SUGGEST MALIGNANT OVARIAN NEOPLASM

- Adnexal mass with thickened, irregularly shaped walls
- Adnexal mass with irregular solid components
- Complex adnexal mass with large cystic component (>10 cm)
- Adnexal cyst with multiple internal septations
- Multiple small, irregular peritoneal lesions representing metastases (peritoneal seeding)
- Ascites
- Peritoneal gelatinous material from pseudomyxoma peritonei suggesting mucin-secreting adenocarcinoma of the ovary

KEY POINTS

1. Ovarian neoplasms are grouped according to the cell type of origin.
2. Primary ovarian neoplasms arise in germ cells, stromal cells, or epithelial cells (75%).
3. Other tumors of the ovaries include lymphoma and metastases from neoplasms of the breasts, uterus, and upper gastrointestinal tumors (Krukenberg tumors).
4. Ovarian neoplasms are often silent until they are at an advanced stage, with 65% of patients having metastatic disease at the time of diagnosis.
5. Patients often present with complaints of weight loss, abdominal distension, pelvic discomfort, or pelvic mass.
6. The most common ultrasonographic finding with ovarian carcinoma is a unilateral, complex adnexal mass.
7. Mixed cystic and solid lesions suggest malignancy and are commonly ovarian cystadenocarcinomas.
8. The presence of ascites increases the probability of malignancy.

■ ENDOMETRIAL CARCINOMA

Anatomy

The uterus normally measures between 6 and 8 cm in length in premenopausal women. In postmenopausal women the uterus may decrease slightly in length to between 4 and 6 cm. The endometrial stripe, referred to as the **endometrial echo complex** (EEC), on ultrasound examination lines the endometrial canal and should measure no more than 14 mm in thickness if the patient is premenopausal or 5 mm if she is postmenopausal. Patients on tamoxifen therapy may have a slightly increased endometrial stripe, but any patient with an EEC greater than 15 mm should undergo further workup to exclude malignancy.

Etiology

The endometrium normally proliferates during the midmenstrual cycle. In postmenopausal women the endometrium becomes atrophic and should not continue to proliferate. Abnormal proliferation of the endometrium may occur because of unopposed estrogen, or it may result from adenocarcinoma or sarcoma.

Epidemiology

Endometrial carcinoma is the most common gynecologic malignancy, with 35,000 new cases per year in the United States. Women in their fifties and sixties are most commonly affected. For the less common endometrial sarcoma, there is a wider range for the age of incidence, between 40 and 60. Risk factors for both are related to increased estrogen states and include early menarche, late menopause, estrogen replacement therapy, obesity, ovulation failure, and nulliparity.

Clinical Manifestations

History

Postmenopausal bleeding is the most common presenting symptom. Other symptoms include vague pelvic pain caused by increasing uterine size.

Physical Examination

Blood in the cervical os is often noted on gynecologic examination. With sarcoma, prolapsing tissue may be seen. The Papanicolaou (Pap) smear may be helpful if it is positive but does not exclude the disease if it is negative. An enlarged uterus or uterine myomas are frequently palpated.

Diagnostic Evaluation

Transvaginal ultrasound is the imaging modality of choice. CT may be helpful in the staging of confirmed cases, but it is not as accurate as MRI. Myomata are frequently visualized with CT and MRI and may be indistinguishable from uterine malignancy. The differential diagnosis in women with postmenopausal bleeding should also include bleeding uterine fibroids, endometrial hyperplasia, endometrial polyps, cervical cancer with bleeding, endometriosis, and side effects of estrogen replacement.

Radiologic Findings

A thickened, echogenic (i.e., bright on ultrasound) endometrial echo complex that measures more than 15 mm in premenopausal women or more than 5 mm in a postmenopausal patient is suggestive of endometrial carcinoma (Figure 7-8). Endometrial hyperplasia or polyps have a similar appearance. An irregular, ill-defined endometrial contour is suspicious for carcinoma. An extension of the echogenic endometrial tissue into or beyond the myometrium is suspicious for malignancy, although adenomyosis (endometriosis of the uterus) may have a similar appearance. CT imaging of endometrial cancer often shows a mass, endometrial enhancement, and fluid within the endometrial canal (Figure 7-9). A dilated canal with fluid may result from a uterine tumor obstructing the internal os of the cervix, cervical cancer, an endometrial polyp, or inflammation at the cervical os. Uterine enlargement is a nonspecific finding that may also be seen with fibroids and adenomyosis.

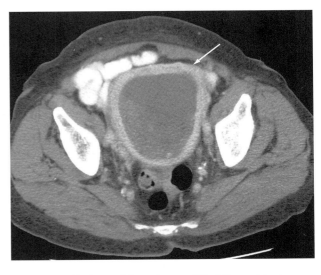

Figure 7-9 • Endometrial carcinoma. CT of the pelvis shows a dilated endometrial cavity with heterogeneous fluid. (Courtesy of Cedars-Sinai Medical Center, Los Angeles, CA.)

KEY POINTS

1. The endometrial stripe, best seen with ultrasound, is the lining of the endometrial canal and should measure no more than 14 mm if the patient is premenopausal or 5 mm if postmenopausal.
2. Postmenopausal bleeding is the most common presenting symptom of endometrial malignancy.
3. Transvaginal ultrasound is the imaging modality of choice.
4. A thickened, irregular, ill-defined endometrial echo complex that measures more than 15 mm (premenopausal) or more than 5 mm (postmenopausal) is highly suggestive of endometrial carcinoma.
5. Fluid within the endometrial canal usually is the result of blood. If the canal is dilated, it suggests an obstructing lesion at the internal os, which may be due to endometrial cancer, cervical cancer, endometrial polyp, or inflammation of the cervical os.

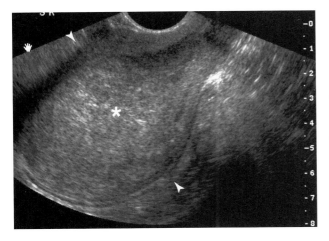

Figure 7-8 • Endometrial carcinoma. Thickened, echogenic endometrium *(asterisk)* on ultrasound of the pelvis. (Walls of the uterus: anterior, *upper arrowhead;* posterior, *lower arrowhead.*) (Courtesy of Cedars-Sinai Medical Center, Los Angeles, CA.)

8 Musculoskeletal Imaging

TRAUMA

▨ COLLES FRACTURE

Anatomy

Radiographic description of fractures follows a systematic approach: First, determine the affected bones and anatomic location of each, for example, the epiphysis, metaphysis, or diaphysis. The diaphysis is divided into proximal, middle, and distal portions. Next describe the pattern of the fracture as simple (two fracture ends, no fragments) or comminuted (more than two fragments). Fracture planes are transverse, oblique, spiral, or longitudinal. Other important features are angulation of the distal fragment, overriding or distracted fragments, and involvement of the growth plate or joint space.

A Colles fracture, by definition, involves the head of the radius with dorsal angulation of the distal fracture fragment. An associated ulnar styloid fracture is present in about 50% of cases.

Etiology

The most common cause is a traumatic fall onto an outstretched hand with the wrist in partial dorsiflexion (Figure 8-1). Force vectors are directed to the distal radius dorsally and proximally.

Epidemiology

The Colles fracture is the most common fracture of the distal forearm. Osteoporosis increases the risk of occurrence, and classically patients are women over age 70 with some degree of osteoporosis.

Clinical Manifestations

History

Patients commonly give a history of a fall while walking. Uneven pavement or misplaced steps frequently cause a person to fall forward and extend the arms in a reflexive action. If a patient cannot recall the cause of the fall, an underlying reason such as ataxia, dehydration, orthostatic hypotension, or syncope should be investigated.

Physical Examination

There is point tenderness over the distal radius and commonly over the ulnar styloid. Soft-tissue swelling is present over the radial aspect of the wrist. The radial pulse should be compared with the contralateral wrist, and sensory and motor functions of the hand should be tested. The median and ulnar nerves and the radial artery are rarely affected, but surgery is required if vascular or neurologic compromise is severe.

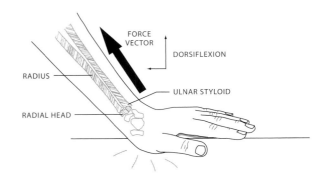

Figure 8-1 · Fall onto outstretched hand and mechanism of Colles fracture.

Diagnostic Evaluation

AP, oblique, and lateral plain radiographs of the distal forearm and wrist are the screening examinations of choice for a patient with a suspected Colles fracture.

Radiologic Findings

Fracture of distal radius with dorsal angulation is the pathognomonic finding for a Colles fracture (Figure 8-2). Typically, a fracture line is seen on the AP view. The lateral view demonstrates the dorsal angulation of the distal radius. Subtle fractures may be detected only as a discontinuity in the normal dense cortical outline. Soft-tissue swelling is an important associated finding that almost always accompanies a fracture. If there is impaction of the radial head, the radius appears foreshortened. An ulnar styloid fracture is seen in about 50% of cases.

A Smith fracture (Figure 8-3) is similar to a Colles fracture, but there is volar rather than dorsal angulation of the distal radial fragment.

KEY POINTS
1. A **Colles fracture** is defined as a fracture of the radial head with dorsal angulation of the distal fragment.
2. Patients give a history of falling onto outstretched hands.

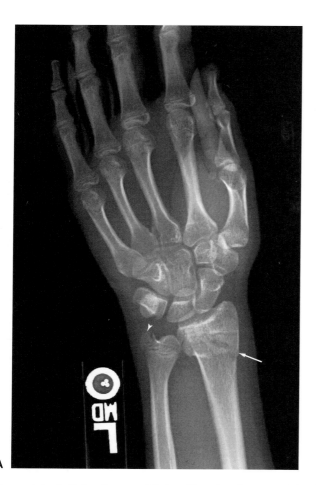

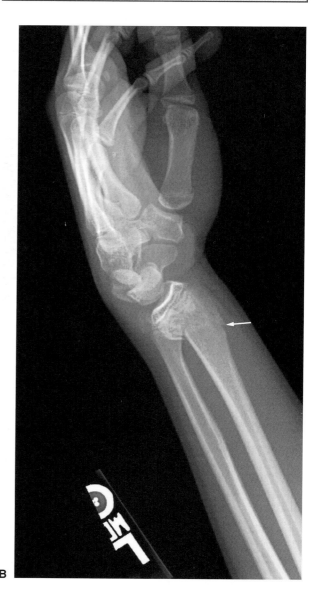

Figure 8-2 • A: Colles fracture, AP view. There is a fracture of the distal radius with mild dorsal angulation of the distal fragment. **B:** Colles fracture, lateral view.
(Courtesy of Cedars-Sinai Medical Center, Los Angeles, CA.)

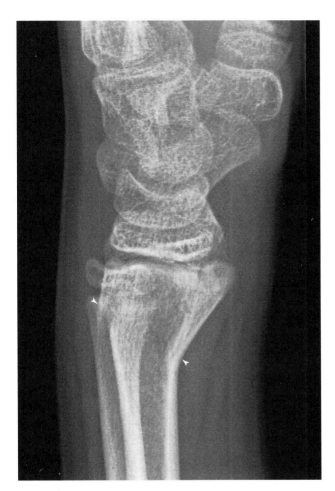

Figure 8-3 • Smith fracture. Fracture of the distal radius with volar angulation of the distal fragment.
(Courtesy of Cedars-Sinai Medical Center, Los Angeles, CA.)

TORUS FRACTURE

Anatomy

A torus or "buckle" fracture may occur in any long bone, but generally it is seen in the radius or tibia.

Etiology

Torus fractures generally occur as a result of "buckling" of the cortex as a result of excessive angulated forces. Trauma, such as jumping from a height greater than 6 feet or a fall onto outstretched hands, may lead to a torus fracture in children aged 5 to 10. Children are susceptible to this type of fracture because the elasticity of their maturing bones causes deformity of

the cortex rather than a fracture along a single plane as in adults.

Clinical Manifestations

History

Generally torus fractures occur after a fall onto an outstretched hand or jumping onto a hard surface from a height of more than 6 feet. This usually happens during sports or during play, such as skateboarding, rollerblading, or bicycling.

Physical Examination

Tenderness to palpations is elicited at the area corresponding to the x-ray findings.

Diagnostic Evaluation

AP, lateral, and oblique radiographs of the affected limb are usually sufficient for the diagnosis. Occasionally radiographs of the contralateral limb are useful for comparison.

Radiologic Findings

The torus or "buckle" fracture is seen as a curved disruption of the cortex and rupture of the periosteum on the convex side, which may extend for a few millimeters up to about 1 cm. The fracture is best seen in profile (Figure 8-4) as opposed to *en face*, and for this reason it is important to obtain three views of the wrist in an attempt to view the fracture at an angle. There is usually mild to moderate overlying soft-tissue swelling and tenderness over the suspected area.

KEY POINTS

1. A torus or "buckle" fracture may occur in any long bone, but generally it is seen in the radius or tibia.
2. The torus fracture commonly occurs in children ages 5 to 10 after a fall onto outstretched hands in the radius or a fall from a height in the tibia.
3. The **torus** refers to the curved disruption of the cortex and periosteum, without a distinct transverse fracture line.

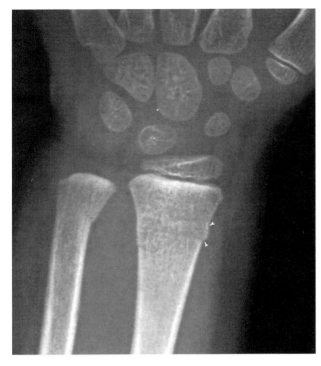

Figure 8-4 • Torus fracture of the distal radius in a 10-year-old child who fell while rollerblading. Notice the buckle in the radial metaphysis on the AP view *(arrowheads)*.
(Courtesy of Cedars-Sinai Medical Center, Los Angeles, CA.)

■ SALTER-HARRIS FRACTURE

Anatomy

The long bones are divided into three sections related to the physis, or growth plate (Figure 8-5). The epi-

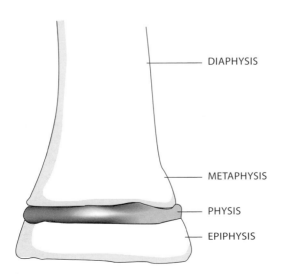

Figure 8-5 • Diagram of the anatomy of bone growth plate.

physis is distal to the physis in the direction of growth; the metaphysis is immediately adjacent to the physis on the opposite side of the epiphysis, and the diaphysis is the long shaft beyond the metaphysis. In growing children with open epiphysial plates, about 35% of all skeletal injuries involve the growth plate in some way. The most common sites are the wrist (50%), ankle (30%), and knee. Damaging the physis can cause growth deformities, such as limb-length discrepancies and angulations.

Etiology

Any trauma with sufficient force can cause a fracture or disruption of the growth plate. The injuries are analogous to ligamentous injuries in adults.

Epidemiology

Growth plate injuries account for about 35% of all skeletal injuries in children between the ages of 10 and 15. Younger children generally will have greenstick (Figure 8-6) or torus (see Figure 8-4) fractures.

Clinical Manifestations

History

Patients present after trauma. In the 10- to 15-year-old age group, this is usually the result of a sports-related injury or a fall. The chief complaint is pain in the affected limb and point tenderness over the fracture.

Physical Examination

Soft-tissue swelling overlying the fracture or diffusely over the affected joint is seen on gross examination. A full neurovascular examination should be performed, as Salter-Harris fractures can affect adjacent nerves or vessels.

Diagnostic Evaluation

AP, lateral, and oblique radiographs of the affected joint are standard for screening of suspected fractures. CT scan of the affected limb may be obtained if intra-articular involvement is suspected but not definite on the plain films. MRI is rarely indicated but may show marrow edema and prove nondisplaced fractures not evident on screening radiographs.

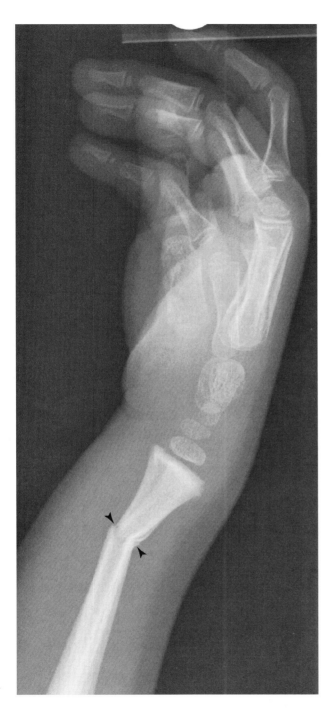

Figure 8-6 • Greenstick fracture of the distal radius and ulna. Only the volar cortices have displaced fractures. The dorsal cortices demonstrate a bending type of fracture.
(Courtesy of Cedars-Sinai Medical Center, Los Angeles, CA.)

Radiologic Findings

Salter-Harris fractures are classified into five types (Figure 8-7). The mnemonic of SALTR describes each type: slipped, above, lower, through, and ruined (Box 8-1).

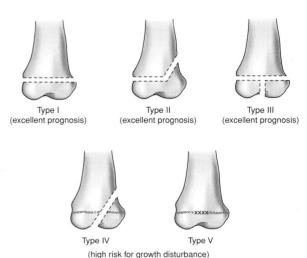

Type I
(excellent prognosis)

Type II
(excellent prognosis)

Type III
(excellent prognosis)

Type IV

Type V

(high risk for growth disturbance)

Figure 8-7 • Epiphyseal fractures: Salter-Harris classification.

BOX 8-1	SALTR MNEMONIC AND CLASSIFICATION

- Type I (5%): "**S**lipped" or displaced physis
- Type II (75%): Fracture **a**bove the physis involving the metaphysis (Figure 8-8)
- Type III (10%): Fracture be**l**ow the physis involving only the epiphysis
- Type IV (10%): Fracture **t**hrough the metaphysis, physis, and epiphysis (Figure 8-9)
- Type V (rare <1%): Crush injury "**r**uined" to the physis

KEY POINTS

1. Salter-Harris fractures are classified into five types. The mnemonic of SALTR describes each type: slipped, above, lower, through, and ruined.
2. These fractures affect children between the ages of 10 and 15.
3. AP, lateral, and oblique radiographs of the affected joint are standard for screening of suspected fractures.

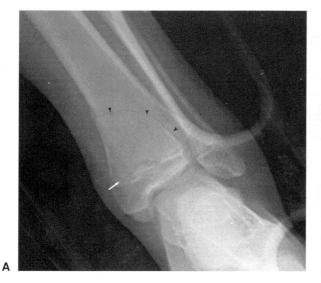

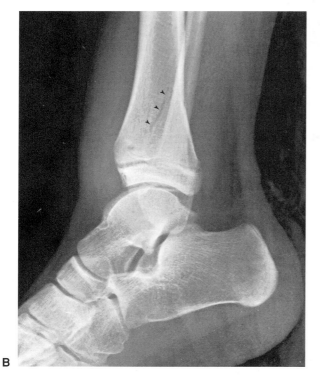

Figure 8-8 • A: AP view of Salter-Harris II fracture of the left ankle in a 12-year-old boy. The fracture line involves the distal tibial metaphysis. **B:** Lateral view of Salter-Harris II fracture in same patient.
(Courtesy of Cedars-Sinai Medical Center, Los Angeles, CA.)

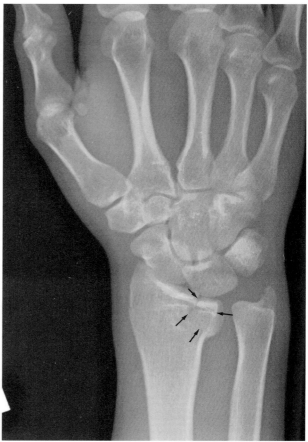

Figure 8-9 • Salter-Harris type IV fracture that extends through the physis in the right radius of a 9-year-old boy.
(Courtesy of Cedars-Sinai Medical Center, Los Angeles, CA.)

▦ HIP FRACTURE

Anatomy

Femoral fractures usually occur at one of three areas: subcapital, intertrochanteric, or subtrochanteric (Figure 8-10). Subtrochanteric fractures are usually associated with more severe trauma and are more common in men. The circumflex artery of the femur, which supplies the femoral head, may be affected, especially with subcapital fractures. Avascular necrosis of the femoral head is a complication of 10% to 30% of subcapital fractures.

Etiology

The underlying etiology is commonly either osteoporosis or chronic systemic steroid use. Acute fractures

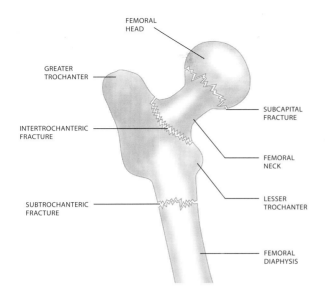

Figure 8-10 • Diagram of common points of femoral fracture.

Diagnostic Evaluation

In addition to the history and physical examination, an AP radiograph of the pelvis and AP and "frog-leg" (abduction and external rotation) lateral views of the affected hip should be obtained. AP and lateral films of the femur and knee may be ordered to exclude other fractures and to exclude other causes of referred pain to the knee. Another important test is the postreduction film, used to exclude fracture fragments not seen on initial films and to confirm adequate fracture reduction to avoid nonunion. If the hip has been also dislocated, a CT should be obtained to exclude any intra-articular osseous fragments post reduction.

Radiologic Findings

Fractures are often seen as a disruption of the cortex, as a lucent fracture line (Figure 8-11), or as an offset of the normal anatomic alignment of the femur if the fracture is displaced. With subcapital fractures, there is often angulation of the femoral head compared with the contralateral side. Nondisplaced fractures may not have any plain film radiographic evidence. For this reason, they are often referred to as **occult fractures.** If the clinical picture is suspicious, but plain films are negative, MRI or radionuclide bone scan is useful. Findings on MRI include linear decreased signal intensity on T1-weighted images, signifying a fracture line. Nuclear scintigraphy is useful after the healing phase begins and radionuclide taken up by osteoblasts demonstrates increased activity, that is, a "hot-spot" on technetium bone scan.

are usually due to trauma, but osteoporotic fractures without associated major trauma have been reported. Pathologic fractures may occur as a result of metastatic lesions or primary bone lesions.

Epidemiology

The incidence of hip fracture is about 200,000 cases per year in the United States. Patients are predominantly postmenopausal women, but men with osteoporosis and any patient taking steroids chronically for other conditions are at increased risk. Inadequate calcium and vitamin D intake, lack of exercise, and alcohol use are predisposing factors.

Clinical Manifestations

History

Pain is noted in the groin area of the affected side. Severe pain is suggestive of a displaced fracture. Patients may complain of pain at rest, but most feel it when attempting to bear weight.

Physical Examination

External rotation and shortening of the affected leg are often noted on gross examination. Pain is elicited on motion of the hip, and referred pain to the knee may be present.

KEY POINTS

1. Fractures of the hip usually occur at one of three places: subcapital, intertrochanteric, and subtrochanteric.
2. Underlying etiology is most commonly osteoporosis attributable to age or chronic use of steroids. Pathologic fractures may occur as a result of metastatic lesions or primary bone lesions.
3. AP radiograph of the pelvis and AP and "frog-leg" lateral views of the affected hip should be obtained.

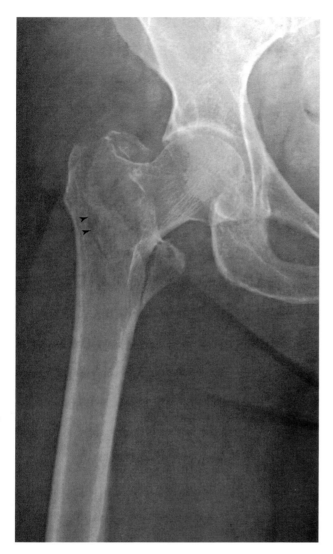

Figure 8-11 • Hip fracture. Intertrochanteric fracture in the right hip of an 83-year-old woman who fell getting out of bed. (Courtesy of Cedars-Sinai Medical Center, Los Angeles, CA.)

▥ RHEUMATOID ARTHRITIS

Etiology

Rheumatoid arthritis is the most common of the inflammatory arthritides. The cause of this disease is still uncertain. There is an association with human leukocyte antigen (HLA) DW4, and environmental factors are also considered.

Epidemiology

The age distribution is from 25 to 55, with a peak in the 20 to 30 range. The ratio of women to men is about 3:1.

Pathogenesis

The underlying pathology is the formation of pannus, the overproduction of synovial tissue, which fills joint spaces and erodes articular cartilage and bone.

Clinical Manifestations

History

Patients' chief complaint is joint pain and stiffness, which is worse in the morning and lasts at least 1 hour.

Physical Examination

Tenderness in the inflamed joints is the most common finding. Symmetric involvement develops with time. Flexion contractures and ulnar deviation at the metacarpophalangeal joint are seen in late stages of disease.

Diagnostic Evaluation

The detection of rheumatoid factor (RF) in the serum is helpful in making the diagnosis, although it is not essential because about 20% of patients may have "seronegative" arthritis, including Reiter syndrome, psoriatic arthritis, and ankylosing spondylitis. Extra-articular manifestations that may aid in the diagnosis include rheumatoid nodules (20% to 25%), vasculitis, scleritis, pericarditis, pleural effusions, and interstitial lung fibrosis.

BOX 8-2	COMMON RADIOLOGIC FINDINGS IN RHEUMATOID ARTHRITIS

- Classic joint deformities, such as swan-neck deformity of the proximal and distal interphalangeal joints of the hands (Figure 8-12), Boutonnière deformity of the phalanges, and ulnar deviation of the wrist
- Periarticular osteopenia (an early finding) and erosions (a late finding) (Figure 8-13)
- Osseous erosions located away from the weight-bearing area of the affected joint
- Uniform joint space narrowing caused by loss of cartilage from invading pannus
- Polyarticular, symmetric joint involvement (metacarpophalangeal, metatarsophalangeal, carpal, tarsal, acromioclavicular, hip, atlantoaxial joints)
- Soft-tissue swelling

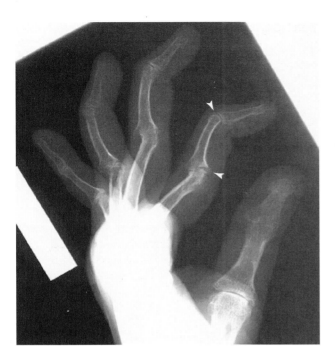

Figure 8-12 • Rheumatoid arthritis. Classic swan-neck deformity of the hands. Hyperextension of the PIP joint and hyperflexion of DIP joint.
(Courtesy of Cedars-Sinai Medical Center, Los Angeles, CA.)

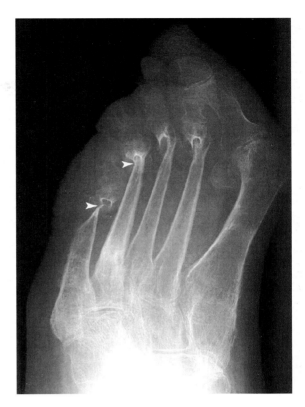

Figure 8-13 • Periarticular erosions in the metatarsal-phalangeal joints.
(Courtesy of Cedars-Sinai Medical Center, Los Angeles, CA.)

Radiologic Findings

PA plain films of the hands and wrists remain the gold standard in both the diagnosis and the follow-up of rheumatoid arthritis. Common radiographic findings are listed in Box 8-2.

KEY POINTS

1. Radiologic diagnosis is made with PA plain films of the hands and wrists.
2. Findings include soft-tissue swelling, periarticular osteopenia, joint space narrowing, and classic deformities of the fingers and wrists.
3. Rheumatoid arthritis is classically bilateral and symmetric.
4. Extra-articular manifestations may aid in the diagnosis.

■ OSTEOMYELITIS

Osteomyelitis refers to inflammation and destruction of bone cortex by infectious agents.

Etiology

Various organisms are implicated in bone infections (bacteria, fungi, mycobacteria). Bone infection can occur either from contiguous spread (from infected adjacent soft tissues, punctures, prostheses, open fractures, etc.) or from hematogenous seeding.

Epidemiology

Patients with diabetes mellitus have high rates of bone infection, particularly in the feet, which can become infected from overlying soft-tissue ulcers. Hematogenous spread is seen in intravenous drug users (gram-negative bacteria) and in ill or immunocompromised patients. *Salmonella* is seen in patients with sickle cell disease (autosplenectomy from repeated infarcts makes them susceptible to encapsulated organisms).

Pathogenesis

Diabetes mellitus results in neuropathy (i.e., pain insensitivity), which can lead to accidental formation

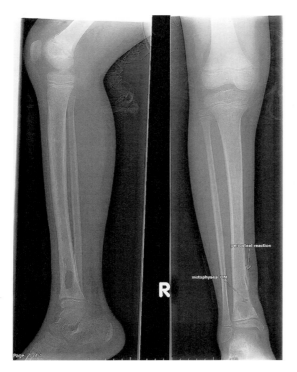

Figure 8-14 • Osteomyelitis. The plain film demonstrates lytic destruction of the distal right tibia, metaphyseal location. Note the cephalad periosteal reaction.
(Courtesy of University of Southern California Medical Center, Los Angeles, CA.)

of ulcers. Children's bones are commonly infected by staphylococci. Osteomyelitis may be complicated by spread into an adjacent joint leading to septic arthritis, which results in rapid erosion of articular cartilage and underlying bone surface.

Clinical Manifestations

History

Patient symptoms include subjective fevers, chills, and pain at the area of infection. Mycobacterial and fungal infections have an indolent course, with symptoms persisting for an extended period, and bone destruction is more severe than the patient's symptoms would indicate.

Physical Examination

Redness, edema, increased local temperature, and tenderness over the area are common findings. Diabetic patients present with infected soft-tissue ulcers.

Diagnostic Evaluation

Acute bacterial osteomyelitis results in inconsistently elevated temperature and white blood cell count. C-reactive protein, a sensitive inflammation marker used by orthopedists routinely, is a reliable test in these cases.

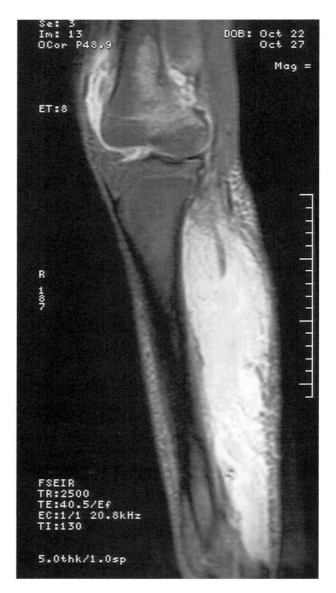

Figure 8-15 • Acute osteomyelitis. Coronal oblique MRI with fat suppression demonstrates high signal intensity within the distal right femur. The fatty marrow suppresses and has a dark signal; the infected area is bright. The bright adjacent soft tissues represent extraosseous extension and joint septic effusion. Debridement of this patient's joints yielded *Fusobacterium*, seeded hematogenously.
(Courtesy of University of Southern California Medical Center, Los Angeles, CA.)

Radiologic Findings

The usual plain-film signs of bone infection are periosteal elevation and lytic cortical lesions (Figure 8-14). These lesions must be distinguished from bone neoplasms, but rapid progression (within days) and peculiar appearance suggest infectious destruction. Chronic bone infection usually results in cortical thickening. It must be kept in mind that plain radiographs are normal until a large portion (i.e., >50%) of bone cortex is destroyed. If clinical suspicion is high, an MRI or a three-phase bone scan is recommended (see Chapter 11).

For spinal involvement, MRI is preferred because it enables visualization of the extension into the spinal canal (i.e., evaluation for cord compression can be performed). Nuclear medicine scans are preferred when multiple sites of infectious seeding are expected (MRI gives good anatomic evaluation, but lengthy imaging is limited to smaller areas, whereas bone scintigraphy can efficiently assess the entire osseous skeleton) (Figure 8-15).

Treatment

Depending on the severity of disease and the extent of bone involvement, prolonged intravenous antibiotic treatment may be instituted. Unfortunately, diabetes mellitus patients have poor blood perfusion to the extremities for good antibiotic penetration and present late because of their neuropathy. In such cases, amputation of the affected bones may be the only treatment.

▩ MALIGNANT BONE NEOPLASMS

Bone tumors may be malignant or benign. The benign bone tumors are too numerous to cover in this chapter. The malignant bone tumors, which are relatively fewer and very important to recognize, are classified as metastatic (more frequent) or primary.

Etiology

Etiology of most osseous malignancies is unknown. Sarcomas are known to arise in the area of prior radiation therapy (i.e., in the cervical vertebrae after radiation therapy for thyroid or other head and neck cancers).

Epidemiology

Malignant primary bone tumors differ in histology in different age groups. First on the list in adults is multiple myeloma, whereas in children and young adults

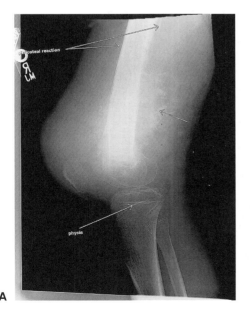
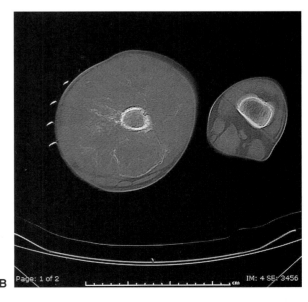

Figure 8-16 • A: Osteosarcoma of the femur. Lateral view of the right knee demonstrates a large mass of the distal femur with deposition of osteoid into the soft tissues *(posterior arrow)*. This tumor was proven at biopsy to be a high-grade osteosarcoma. **B:** CT scan with bone windowing performed on the same patient demonstrates the "sunburst" appearance of osteosarcoma. (Courtesy of University of Southern California Medical Center, Los Angeles, CA.)

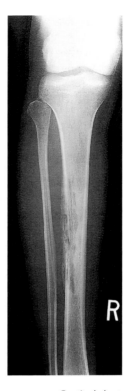

Figure 8-17 • Ewing sarcoma. Cortical destruction of mid right tibia with cephalad and caudad periosteal reaction was proven by pathology to be caused by Ewing sarcoma. In the long bones, sometimes this neoplasm may be difficult to distinguish from osteomyelitis based on radiographic findings alone. Note the bandage artifact overlying the soft tissues.
(Courtesy of University of Southern California Medical Center, Los Angeles, CA.)

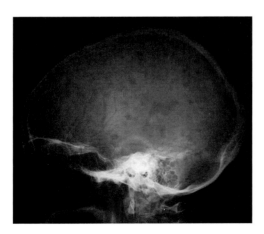

Figure 8-18 • Lateral skull in multiple myeloma showing widespread well-defined "punched-out" lytic lesions in the cranial vault.
(Reprinted with permission from Patel, R. Lecture Notes: Radiology, 2nd ed. Figure 7.16, p. 190, Malden, MA: Blackwell Publishing, 2005.)

it is osteosarcoma. Sarcomas are the most common primary bone malignancy between ages 10 to 25, with male preponderance. Ewing sarcoma is attributed to a chromosomal translocation (11,22).

The metastatic bone tumors span the whole age spectrum, from infants to older adults. In children and adolescents, leukemia and lymphoma are common. For adults, other metastatic tumors also should be considered (lung, breast, prostate, etc.).

Pathogenesis

The sclerotic (dense) bone lesions are related to increased osteoid formation. The bone lysis is due to replacement of bone by tumor or by stimulation of osteoclast-activating factor secreted by the plasma cells (as in multiple myeloma).

Clinical Manifestations

History

Patients present either with a mass or with pain in the involved area. Many patients erroneously temporally relate the onset of symptoms with trauma.

Physical Examination

Tenderness may sometimes be elicited on palpation and a mass is found.

Diagnostic Evaluation

When an osteosarcoma is suspected on the basis of plain films (Figure 8-16A), an MRI of the involved bone should be performed to identify any additional areas, called **skip lesions**. A CT scan of the chest should be performed to evaluate for pulmonary metastases because sarcomas are known to spread hematogenously. At times metastases of sarcomas may occur at other sites, and a bone scan is recommended to rule out their presence. In children, multiple sarcomas may occur at different locations (osteosarcomatosis).

Multiple myeloma is worked up with a skeletal survey (evaluation of all bones by plain film) because the bone scan will be negative (no radioactive tracer is taken up as no osteoblastic activity is present in these bone lesions).

Metastatic bone involvement by extraosseous tumors is preferentially imaged by nuclear medicine bone scintigraphy (see Chapter 11).

Radiologic Findings

A stereotypical description of periosteal reaction (encountered on board examinations) for osteosarcoma is termed "sunburst" (Figure 8-16 B) and for Ewing sarcoma, an "onion skin" (Figure 8-17) appearance.

Multiple myeloma is one of the lytic bone lesions, and involvement of multiple bones and skull lesions makes this diagnosis a more certain conclusion. The skull lesions' appearance has been described as "punched out" (Figure 8-18).

The metastatic bone lesions are classified as blastic and lytic. Certain metastases are known for associated increased osteoid formation, with high density seen on x-ray (breast, prostate), whereas others are almost always lytic (e.g., as in renal cell carcinoma).

Treatment

Biopsy of bone lesions has to be done with the recommendation of the orthopedic surgeon because the biopsy tract is considered contaminated by a malignant tumor, and it has to be carefully excised at surgery. The biopsy is preferably done by a musculoskeletal radiologist, under CT guidance, for good localization and yield (biopsy should be taken from the cellular tumor periphery, not from the necrotic core). Depending on the severity of the appendicular sarcoma, a limb-salvage excision or an amputation is performed. If the neurovascular bundle is involved, an amputation is the choice. In high-grade tumors, a chemotherapy protocol is also implemented.

For multiple myeloma and osseous metastases, chemotherapy is the treatment, sometimes with additional palliative radiation therapy.

KEY POINTS

1. Many patients erroneously relate the development symptoms with trauma.
2. If an osteosarcoma is suspected on plain film, an MRI of the extremity should be ordered to look for additional lesions in the area (skip lesions).
3. A CT scan of the chest should be ordered in patients with osteosarcoma because hematogenously spread pulmonary metastases are common.
4. The study of choice in osseous metastases is bone scan; in multiple myeloma, it is the skeletal survey (plain films of central and appendicular skeleton).
5. Bone metastases are lytic (i.e., they cause bone destruction) or blastic (i.e., they stimulate osteoid deposition).

Pediatric Imaging

■ FOREIGN-BODY ASPIRATION

Anatomy

A foreign body that is aspirated into the airway is usually a small object (most commonly a small piece of food, a peanut, a coin, or a small toy) that is inhaled rather than swallowed. Normally the epiglottis prevents aspiration by covering the laryngeal vestibule and diverting food into the esophagus. Sites of obstruction are almost exclusively the lower lobe bronchi, most commonly on the right because the right mainstem bronchus has a nearly vertical course and a larger caliber.

Etiology

In the normal course of development, children aged 1 to 3 years tend to investigate objects by placing them in their mouths. Developmentally this is a vulnerable time because they may aspirate the object into the airway when inhaling normally.

Epidemiology

Children younger than age 3 are most susceptible to foreign-body aspiration because they tend to play with small objects and frequently place them in their mouths. Toys should be inspected for small, removable parts. Coins, keys, stones, and foods such as nuts and peas should be avoided because of their small size and frequent association with airway obstruction.

Pathogenesis

Acute obstruction of the airway prevents oxygenation of the affected lung. Without airflow, the obstructed portion of lung will collapse. Chronic obstruction leads to pneumonia and bronchiectasis.

Clinical Manifestations

History

Children often present with sudden onset of wheezing, choking, or respiratory distress while playing or eating. With partial obstruction, they are able to cough and often have acute wheezing. In complete obstruction, they may have shortness of breath, tachypnea, and hypoxemia. If the obstruction is prolonged, loss of consciousness may result from the oxygen deprivation.

Physical Examination

On auscultation, there is often absent or decreased breath sounds on the side of the obstruction. Use of accessory muscles of respiration is noted as the child struggles to aerate the lungs. Grunting and wheezing are common. The oropharynx should be inspected in an attempt to visualize the obstructing object, which potentially could be removed. Oxygen saturation on pulse oximetry is reduced.

Diagnostic Evaluation

When a foreign-body airway obstruction is suspected, the primary screening study is the frontal CXR with right and left decubitus views. Fluoroscopic examination of the lungs may be performed if the radiographs are equivocal. CT of the chest is not typically performed but may be helpful in demonstrating the object if coronal reformations are included. Direct visualization with endoscopy may be needed because up to 30% of cases with negative radiologic findings turn out to be positive.

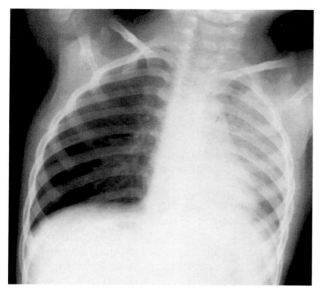

Figure 9-1 • Foreign-body aspiration. Hyperlucency of the right lung on expiration. The left lung has compressive changes normal for an expiratory film. This patient had a peanut in the right mainstem bronchus.
(Courtesy of Cedars-Sinai Medical Center, Los Angeles, CA.)

Radiologic Findings

With bronchial obstruction, the most common finding is hyperlucency of the lung on the affected side as a result of air trapping (Figure 9-1). The obstructing object acts as a ball valve, allowing air to enter the lung but not to escape. On decubitus views, the lung on the side on which the patient is lying is more collapsed than the nondependent lung. When both decubitus views are obtained, the lung with the obstruction remains hyperinflated on both views (Figure 9-2 A, B). Atelectasis of all or part of the lung distal to the obstruction may be seen, although it is less common in bronchial obstruction.

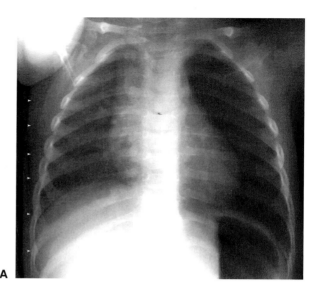

A

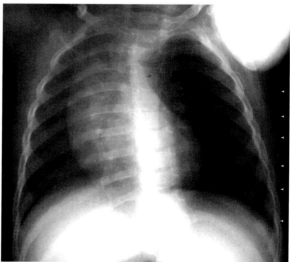

B

Figure 9-2 • A: Foreign-body aspiration. Right lateral decubitus view of the chest shows that the right lung compresses normally when it is dependent (A). Compare with left lateral decubitus view (B). **B:** Left lateral decubitus view shows the left lung remains hyperinflated, although it is the dependent lung (*arrowheads* point to dependent side). This indicates a left mainstem bronchus foreign body. The patient inhaled a small plastic building block.
(Courtesy of Cedars-Sinai Medical Center, Los Angeles, CA.)

KEY POINTS

1. Airway obstruction occurs most commonly in children ages one to three years.
2. Presenting symptoms are sudden onset of choking, gagging, or coughing.
3. The most common radiologic finding is hyperlucency and hyperinflation of the lung on the affected side due to air trapping.

In upper airway obstruction of the larynx or trachea, the CXR may appear normal or with bilateral hyperinflation of the lungs.

■ RESPIRATORY DISTRESS SYNDROME

Anatomy

Respiratory distress syndrome (RDS) is the most common cause of respiratory distress in neonates. In the normal lung, the alveoli are coated with a surfactant that prevents the airspaces from collapsing during expiration. In RDS the alveoli are poorly formed and collapsed, not allowing the proper exchange of oxygen with the bloodstream.

Etiology

RDS, also known as **hyaline membrane disease,** is caused by a deficiency in alveolar surfactant. Type II pneumocytes begin producing surfactant at 24 weeks' gestational age, and peak production occurs at 36 weeks. Without surfactant, surface tension within alveoli increases and atelectasis occurs during expiration. Increasing inspiratory pressures are required to expand the alveoli.

Epidemiology

The risk of RDS correlates with prematurity of the neonate. Fifty percent of all newborns born at 28 weeks' gestation will have RDS. The incidence decreases as the gestational age increases. For term infants, the incidence is less than 5%. For this reason, RDS should be high on the differential diagnosis for premature neonates and low for full-term infants.

Pathogenesis

The surfactant deficiency results in collapsed alveoli, decreased oxygenation, and pulmonary vasoconstriction. This leads in turn to capillary damage and leakage of plasma into the alveoli, which combines with fibrin and necrotic pneumocytes to form the proteinaceous material called **hyaline membranes** in the airspaces. The hyaline membranes prevent oxygen from diffusing across the alveolar membrane, leading to further hypoxemia and respiratory distress.

Clinical Manifestations

History

The onset of increasing dyspnea and hypoxia 1 to 2 hours after birth is the most common presentation. Usually the infant is intubated due to increasing oxygen requirement.

Physical Examination

Tachypnea, grunting, nasal flaring, chest retractions, and cyanosis are noted within the first 2 hours after birth. Breath sounds are decreased bilaterally because of poor air entry.

Diagnostic Evaluation

If the history and physical findings are consistent with RDS, arterial blood gas sampling should be performed to determine the severity of hypoxemia. A stat chest radiograph is obtained to exclude pneumonia, pneumothorax, or other causes of respiratory distress in the newborn. Intubation and mechanical ventilation are often necessary. If RDS is indeed the cause, the infant will eventually require mechanical ventilation.

Radiologic Findings

RDS is suspected in a premature infant with any opacification in the lungs. Diagnosis cannot be based on a single CXR, especially if the infant is not intubated. Diffuse "ground-glass" or reticulogranular opacifications are most common (Figure 9-3). Low lung volumes are often present initially, especially before intubation is done. Follow-up films often reveal progression to air trapping with pulmonary interstitial

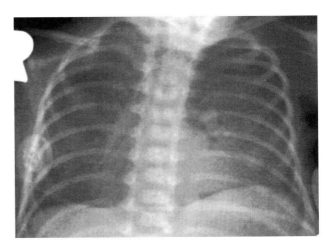

Figure 9-3 • Respiratory distress syndrome. This PA chest radiograph reveals low lung volumes and diffuse ground-glass opacification in a premature infant born at 30 weeks' gestation. (Courtesy of Cedars-Sinai Medical Center, Los Angeles, CA.)

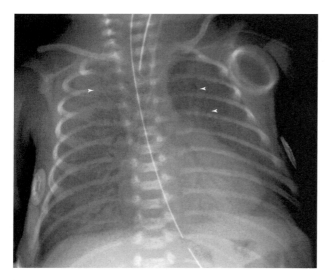

Figure 9-4 • Respiratory distress syndrome. This patient is intubated, and there are diffuse ground-glass opacifications consistent with RDS. Subtle tortuous lucencies represent pulmonary interstitial emphysema *(arrowheads)*.
(Courtesy of Cedars-Sinai Medical Center, Los Angeles, CA.)

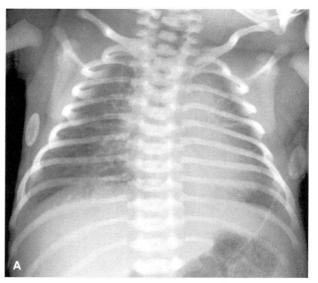

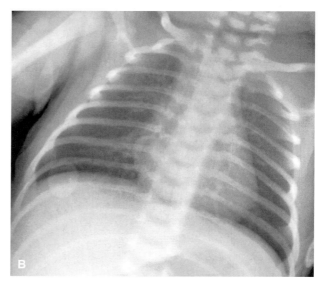

emphysema (Figure 9-4), an accumulation of gas in the peribronchial spaces, and increasing diffuse opacities approaching whiteout of the lungs. The differential diagnosis includes pneumonia, pulmonary edema, and transient tachypnea of the newborn (Figure 9-5), a condition in which there is residual pulmonary fluid and that gradually clears after 2 to 3 days. Complications of RDS include pneumothorax (Figure 9-6A, B) and pneumomediastinum (Figure 9-6C) resulting from decreased compliance of the alveoli and the high pulmonary pressures needed to oxygenate the patients.

KEY POINTS

1. RDS, also known as **hyaline membrane disease,** is caused by a deficiency in alveolar surfactant.
2. The risk of RDS increases with increasing prematurity of the neonate.
3. Diffuse ground-glass or reticulonodular opacifications are most common.

Figure 9-5 • **A:** Transient tachypnea of the newborn. Chest radiograph of a full-term infant reveals diffuse parenchymal opacification. **B:** Follow-up film of patient in (A) taken 3 days later reveals that the diffuse parenchymal opacification has cleared.
(Courtesy of Cedars-Sinai Medical Center, Los Angeles, CA.)

traverses back to the left and the ligament of Treitz is normally left of the midline.

■ DUODENAL STENOSIS

Anatomy

The C-loop of the duodenum normally lies posterior and to the right of the pylorus of the stomach. It

Etiology

Duodenal stenosis is caused by a failure of recanalization of the duodenum during embryologic development, which normally occurs at 10 weeks' gestation.

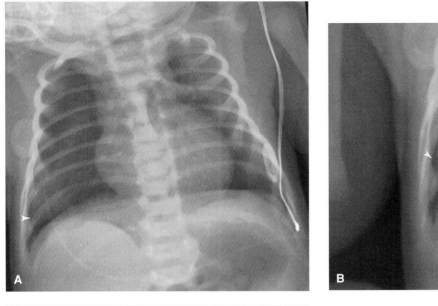

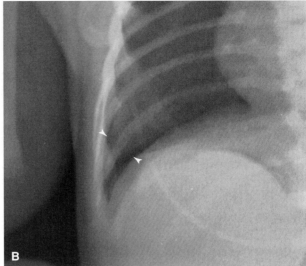

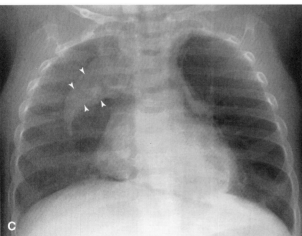

Figure 9-6 • A: Pneumothorax. An area of lucency is seen in the right lower thorax near the right costophrenic angle. **B:** Magnification view of (A). This was a complication of long-standing RDS. **C:** Pneumomediastinum. Patient had been intubated for RDS and developed pneumomediastinum from barotrauma. Note elevation of the right portion of the thymus, a finding commonly called the "sail sign."
(Courtesy of Cedars-Sinai Medical Center, Los Angeles, CA.)

Epidemiology

The incidence is about 1:3500 live births. There is a 30% association of duodenal atresia and Down syndrome. Duodenal stenosis and atresia commonly manifest within 24 hours of birth.

Clinical Manifestations

History

Classically the history is a newborn with bilious vomiting and an inability to tolerate feeding because of the obstruction. The vomiting is nonprojectile compared

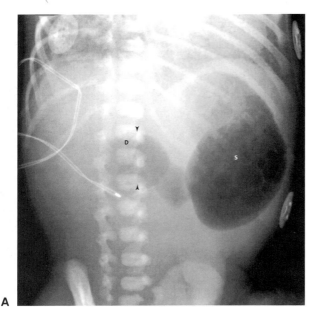
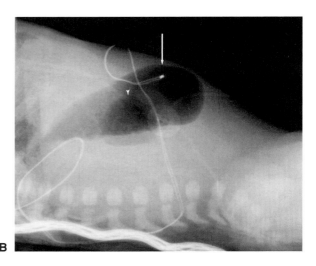

A **B**

Figure 9-7 • **A:** Duodenal stenosis. AP radiograph of the abdomen of a child who presented with bilious vomiting. The image reveals a classic "double-bubble" sign *(arrowhead)*, which represents the stomach (S) and the duodenal bulb (D), filled with gas and secretions. **B:** Duodenal stenosis. Cross-table lateral view reveals gas in the stomach *(arrow)* that is anterior to the duodenal bulb *(arrowhead)*, also filled with gas. Notice that there is a paucity of gas in the rest of the abdomen.
(Courtesy of Cedars-Sinai Medical Center, Los Angeles, CA.)

with pyloric stenosis, which presents with nonbilious projectile vomiting after each feeding.

Physical Examination

Abdominal distension, which represents the distended stomach, is often noted; frequently, however, the examination is normal. Imperforate anus is associated with a small percentage of cases.

Diagnostic Evaluation

The diagnosis is suspected clinically, and a plain radiograph of the abdomen should be obtained.

Radiologic Findings

The classic finding is the "double-bubble" sign, which represents the dilated stomach and duodenal bulb (Figure 9-7). Because air cannot pass beyond the duodenum, there is a paucity of bowel gas throughout the abdomen.

Differential Diagnosis

The differential diagnosis of a "double-bubble" sign on an abdominal radiograph includes duodenal atresia, duodenal stenosis, annular pancreas, and midgut volvulus.

KEY POINTS

1. Duodenal atresia is caused by failure of recanalization of the duodenum during embryologic development.
2. There is a 30% association of duodenal atresia and Down syndrome.
3. The history is a newborn with bilious nonprojectile vomiting.
4. The classic radiologic finding is the "double-bubble" sign.

■ MECONIUM ASPIRATION

Etiology

Meconium is the sterile intestinal material of the newborn. It contains mucosal epithelial cells, bile, and mucus. Normally meconium is passed from the rectum within 12 hours of delivery. Meconium aspiration occurs when the meconium is passed in utero and mixes with the amniotic fluid. Risk factors include postmaturity (42 weeks' gestational age), fetal distress from prolonged labor, premature rupture of membranes, and congenital infection.

Epidemiology

Passing of meconium into the amniotic fluid occurs in about 10% of all live births and usually is associated with postterm gestations. Clinically significant meconium aspiration occurs in 10% of these infants, or about 1% of all live births.

Pathogenesis

It is believed that fetal hypoxia from any of the causes listed above triggers a vagal nerve-mediated expulsion of meconium from the GI tract into the amniotic fluid. The aspirated meconium acts as a chemical irritant in the lungs and causes an inflammatory response that varies from mild to severe, depending on the amount of aspiration.

Clinical Manifestations

History

Green-colored meconium is noted at birth, especially during suctioning of the neonate's airway. Sometimes the aspiration is undetected at birth but suspected when the patient manifests tachypnea and hypoxia.

Physical Examination

Diffuse, coarse rales are heard on auscultation. The newborn may have an oxygen requirement that increases as the chemical pneumonitis causes an increased inflammatory reaction.

Diagnostic Evaluation

The chest radiograph is the diagnostic imaging study of choice. Fever should be monitored, blood cultures drawn to exclude infection, and blood gas taken to determine the extent of hypoxemia. Serial daily CXRs are obtained until there are signs of resolution. Radiographs commonly worsen over the first few days but in most cases begin to clear by 5 days.

Radiologic Findings

The most common finding is diffuse patchy opacification of the lungs. The pattern is often described as

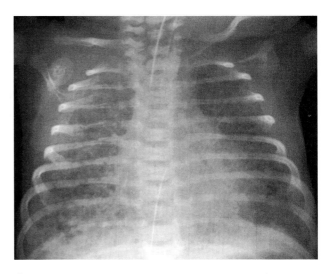

Figure 9-8 • Meconium aspiration. AP chest radiograph reveals coarse opacifications of the lungs bilaterally.
(Courtesy of Cedars-Sinai Medical Center, Los Angeles, CA).

"coarse" because of filling of the airspaces with meconium and the surrounding inflammatory reaction (Figure 9-8). The lungs are often hyperinflated, and air in bronchograms is commonly seen. Pneumothoraces develop as the meconium causes ball-valve obstruction of airways.

KEY POINTS

1. Meconium aspiration occurs when the meconium is passed in utero and mixes with the amniotic fluid.
2. Meconium acts as a chemical irritant in the lungs and causes an inflammatory response.
3. The chest radiograph should be the first imaging study performed.
4. The most common finding is diffuse coarse opacification of the lungs.

■ INTUSSUSCEPTION

Anatomy

Bowel peristalsis leads to invagination and telescoping of a segment of proximal bowel (intussusceptum) into a more distal segment (intussuscepiens). The most common location is at the ileocolic area.

Etiology

Most cases are idiopathic (i.e., about 90%). This condition is suspected to be a result of viral-induced hyperplasia of the intestinal lymphoid tissue (Peyer patches). A minority of intussusception cases are caused by a "leading point" (e.g., Meckel's diverticulum, polyp, tumors, lipomas, or parasites). Involvement of bowel with lymphoma as well as edema of the bowel wall resulting from hematomas caused by Henoch-Schönlein purpura can manifest with intussusception.

Epidemiology

Idiopathic intussusception occurs at an early age (between a few months and 2 years of age). The older the child is, the higher the clinical suspicion for an underlying pathology.

Clinical Manifestations

History

In infants pain is less severe than in older children. Crampy, intermittent abdominal pain, with alternate episodes of comfort, is the most common presentation. Vomiting and "currant-jelly stools" can occur.

Physical Examination

An abdominal mass may be palpable on examination.

Diagnostic Evaluation

The diagnostic examination and concomitant therapy of choice should be a fluoroscopy-guided air or water-soluble contrast (hypaque) pressure enema. Barium is not used because surgical intervention may be necessary and the barium would interfere in the surgical field (and theoretically can cause peritonitis). The enemas are more likely to be successful in an ileocolic intussusception than in an ileoileal intussusception because good pressure buildup is easier to resolve when it is closer to the rectum.

Before an enema is started, a plain film of the abdomen should exclude bowel perforation (pneumoperitoneum), and peritonitis should not be present. The child should be administered prophylactic IV antibiotics before the procedure in case of iatrogenic perforation.

If an air enema is chosen, a needle should be prepared for rapid evacuation of a tension pneumoperitoneum in case perforation occurs. A manometer is attached to the insufflator to ensure that the intraluminal pressure does not become too high (>120 mm Hg).

Water-soluble contrast is introduced per rectum under gravity with fluoroscopic guidance. The contrast bag should be hung about 3 feet above the fluoroscopy table.

Three technically well-performed attempts (contrast or air is seen at the intussusception, and pressure is maintained for 3 minutes) are recommended before aborting the procedure. If the enema is successful at reducing the intussusception, but recurrences occur, an additional two enemas are allowed before surgical intervention.

Radiologic Findings

The initial plain radiograph may show a mass outlined by colonic gas (Figure 9-9). Paucity of bowel gas can also be present if gas has passed from the colon. Small-bowel dilatation or obstruction just proximal to the intussusception also may be noted. During the enema, an abrupt cutoff of air or contrast progression occurs at the intussusception site (Figure 9-10). A "coil spring" appearance is described as gas outlines the invaginated bowel. When reduction is successful, the air or the contrast progresses freely proximally into the small bowel.

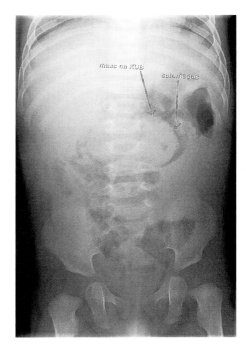

Figure 9-9 • Plain radiograph of the abdomen shows a midabdominal ovoid mass outlined by colon gas. This finding, correlated with the clinical presentation, is pathognomonic for intussusception.
(Courtesy of University of Southern California Medical Center, Los Angeles, CA.)

KEY POINTS

1. The abdominal plain radiograph in cases of intussusception has to be obtained to rule out pneumoperitoneum. The abdominal film is not normal, but the findings can be nonspecific (the intussusception mass can be seen, but sometimes the only clue is paucity of colonic bowel gas).

2. The high-pressure enema should be performed in agreement with the pediatric surgeon, and certain precautions are mandatory: prepare for inadvertent perforation, and administer prophylactic antibiotics.

3. If the intussusception is recalcitrant or the child is older than 2 years of age, surgical intervention may help to elucidate the cause of intussusception (e.g., a neoplasm such as lymphoma).

4. Intussusception is a serious condition that requires timely action to prevent bowel necrosis.

Ultrasound can also be used for diagnosis and will show a mass with a transverse-plane appearance of alternate hyperechoic (fat) and hypoechoic rings representing the telescoped bowel segment. Ultrasound is limited by the operator's skill, and images may be hindered by bowel gas (echogenic). Although CT shows an intussusception well, this modality uses a high dose of radiation that is better avoided in pediatric patients.

■ VESICOURETERAL REFLUX

Etiology

Vesicoureteral reflux is attributed mainly to an abnormally wide angle of insertion of the ureters into the

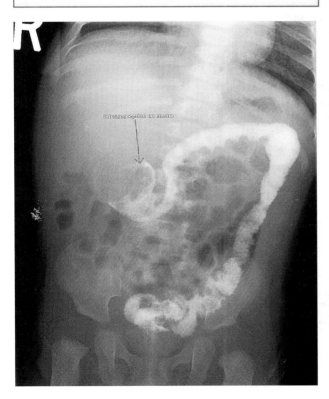

Figure 9-10. • Contrast enema demonstrates midtransverse colon and a lack of progression of contrast toward the hepatic flexure. The intraluminal filling defect represents the intussusception. This radiograph was taken with the colon decompressed (some of the initially introduced contrast has been evacuated).
(Courtesy of University of Southern California Medical Center, Los Angeles, CA.)

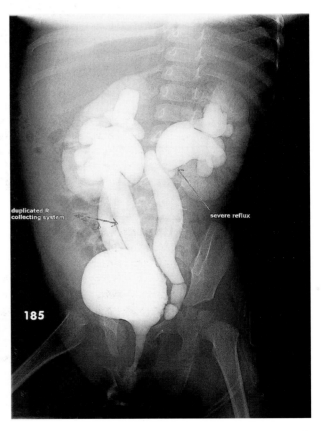

Figure 9-11 • Severe (grade V) vesicoureteral reflux. Single, slightly oblique view from voiding cystourethrogram shows contrast refluxing from the urinary bladder into the ureters, extending intrarenally (the renal parenchyma is outlined by contrast). This patient also has a duplicated right renal collecting system (two right ureters).
(Courtesy of University of Southern California Medical Center, Los Angeles, CA.)

urinary bladder trigone. A high percentage (about 80%) of children outgrow this anomaly as growth changes the ureteral insertion angle. Boys are also affected by posterior urethral valves resulting in urethral obstruction. Ectopic insertion of the ureter and urinary bladder anatomic (diverticula) or functional (neurogenic bladder) anomalies also predispose to reflux.

Epidemiology

Girls are more commonly affected than boys are, but only boys have posterior urethral valves. African American children are least often affected by vesicureteral reflux.

Clinical Manifestations

History

Children present with a variety of symptoms of urinary tract infection (e.g., dysuria, fever, abdominal pain, urinary frequency).

Physical Examination

All girls with recurrent infections or pyelonephritis and all boys require radiographic workup for urinary tract anomalies.

Diagnostic Evaluation

The diagnosis of vesicoureteral reflux is imperative because antibiotic prophylaxis against urinary tract infection needs to be instituted. It is thought that sterile urine reflux does not cause significant renal damage but infected urine causes renal scarring. It is also important to evaluate the degree of vesicoureteral reflux because less severe cases (grades I through III) can be managed conservatively and usually resolve spontaneously, whereas grades IV and V require surgical ureteral reimplantation.

The studies of choice are the voiding cystourethrogram (VCUG) or the radionuclide cystogram. The VCUG is the preferred study if delineation of the anatomy is necessary, but the radiation exposure is

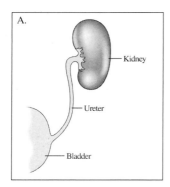

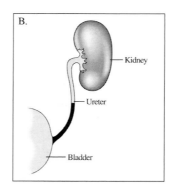

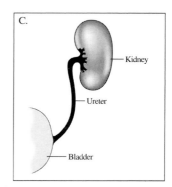

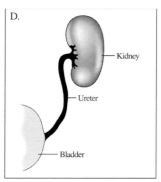

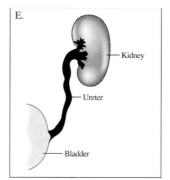

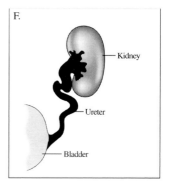

Figure 9-12 • Grading of vesicoureteral reflux. **(A)** Normal. **(B)** Grade I vesicoureteral reflux: Urine refluxes part-way up the ureter. **(C)** Grade II: Urine refluxes all the way up the ureter. **(D)** Grade III: Urine refluxes all the way up the ureter, with dilation of the ureter and calyces (part of the kidney where urine collects). **(E)** Grade IV: Urine refluxes all the way up the ureter, with marked dilation of the ureter and calyces. **(F)** Grade V: Massive reflux of urine up the ureter, with marked tortuosity and dilation of the ureter and calyces.
(Reprinted with permission from Zaslau, S. *Blueprints Urology*, Figure 10.1, p. 113. Malden, MA: Blackwell Publishing, 2005).

significantly higher. For this reason, in boys a VCUG is usually chosen to evaluate for posterior urethral valves as the cause of vesicoureteral reflux. A VCUG is performed by catheterizing the child and instilling contrast into the urinary bladder. The child is then allowed to void on the fluoroscopy table while fluoroscopic imaging is performed to capture any reflux that may occur only during micturition.

The renal nuclear cystogram also involves catheterization and instillation of a radiotracer into the urinary bladder. The child is placed on the gamma camera, and imaging is obtained before, during, and after voiding to ensure reflux capture.

Ultrasound is the preferred modality in pediatric patients because it does not involve ionizing radiation. However, in cases of suspected vesicoureteral reflux, a negative ultrasound is insufficient because the urinary system is not continuously under pressure and the reflux can occur intermittently, for short periods, and sometimes only during voiding. However, ultrasound can evaluate for hydronephrosis, ureteroceles (invagination of ureter within the urinary bladder), or bladder diverticula.

Radiologic Findings

During a VCUG, contrast is seen refluxing from the urinary bladder into the ureters (Figure 9-11), and various degrees exist (from grade I [mild] to V [the most severe]) (Figure 9-12). Similar findings can be documented by radionuclide cystography. If the vesicoureteral reflux is due to posterior urethral valves, an abrupt transition between a dilated proximal urethra and a normal-caliber distal urethra is identified at fluoroscopy.

KEY POINTS

1. Radiographic evaluation for urinary tract anomalies is recommended in children with urinary tract infections (particularly all boys) because medical (antibiotic prophylaxis) or surgical treatment, depending on the severity of the anomaly, must be instituted for vesicoureteral reflux.
2. A VCUG uses fluoroscopy and plain film to document reflux and provides superior anatomic detail, but it uses a significantly higher dose of radiation than the radionuclide cystography.
3. Careful imaging must be performed because the vesicoureteral reflux may be subtle or intermittent, and it may occur only during micturition.

Interventional Radiology

GENERAL PRINCIPLES

Interventional radiology encompasses the use of various imaging modalities to guide the performance of procedures. Fluoroscopy, ultrasound, CT, and even MRI can be used to direct needles and catheters for biopsies and aspirations or to place indwelling devices, such as catheters, stents, or filters. The types of procedures performed by the interventional radiology service differ from institution to institution, but this chapter touches on a broad range of these services.

Interventional procedures can be both diagnostic and therapeutic. Angiography involves the administration of iodinated contrast through the intravascular system to provide a picture under fluoroscopy of the arterial anatomy. Under certain circumstances, if a vascular abnormality is seen, various devices can be advanced through the vessels to provide therapeutic measures. For example, a bleeding vessel can be embolized, or a stenotic vessel can be dilated with a balloon or propped open with an indwelling stent. Needles and catheters can also be advanced percutaneously under ultrasound or fluoroscopic guidance into the renal collecting system or the biliary system to perform antegrade nephrostograms or percutaneous transhepatic cholangiography as diagnostic procedures. A catheter can be left in the renal collecting system to drain urine continually if a patient's ureter is obstructed, in which case it would be called a **nephrostomy tube.** One left in the biliary system would be termed a **percutaneous biliary drainage catheter.**

An important element of any procedure is obtaining informed consent from the patient. The exact nature of a procedure, as well as the risks, benefits, and alternatives, must be clearly explained to a patient before the procedure begins. This discussion with the patient must be documented, and a record must be placed in the patient's chart. It is also important to review a patient's most recent laboratory values, including prothrombin time (PT), partial thromboplastin time (PTT), international normalized ratio (INR), and platelets to evaluate for any coagulopathy; blood urea nitrogen (BUN) and creatinine levels if contrast is going to be administered; and any other laboratory values relevant to the patient's medical condition.

It is important to maintain a sterile environment during the performance of any procedure that involves interruption of the skin, an important barrier to infection. Similar to the sterile environment in a surgical suite, various measures must be taken to minimize the chance of introducing an infectious agent into the patient. These measures include the use of gloves and other equipment that has been sterilized. Once a sterile environment has been ensured, it is essential to avoid any physical contact between sterile and nonsterile materials. Once there has been such contact, the involved item can no longer be considered sterile and must not be used within the sterile field.

A common technique used to gain access percutaneously is called the Seldinger technique. A hollow needle is initially placed under fluoroscopic, CT, or ultrasound guidance, with the tip of the needle in the desired location. A guidewire is then advanced through the needle. Holding the wire in place, the needle is then removed and a catheter is placed over the wire; then the wire is removed, leaving the catheter in the desired location.

Interventional radiology is a rapidly growing and changing field. It is, of course, impossible to touch even briefly on many of the common procedures that are performed. This chapter is intended to provide a cross-section of some of the most commonly performed procedures.

■ THORACIC AORTIC ANEURYSM

Anatomy

The thoracic aorta begins at the aortic valves and traditionally ends at the diaphragmatic hiatus. It is usually divided into three parts: the ascending aorta, the aortic arch, and the descending aorta. The arch begins at the origin of the brachiocephalic artery (also known as the **innominate artery**) and includes the origins of the left common carotid and the left subclavian arteries. The division between the arch and the descending aorta is the ligamentum arteriosum, which is distal to the left subclavian artery.

A patient's age and the location and the morphology of the aneurysm can be important clues to the etiology of an aneurysm. Among ascending aortic aneurysms, atherosclerosis is the most common cause for older patients. Inflammatory disease and collagen vascular diseases are more common in younger patients. Takayasu arteritis can cause fusiform ascending aortic aneurysms. Marfan syndrome is associated with aortic valve dilatation and effacement of the sinotubular ridge. Syphilitic aneurysms spare the sinotubular junction and often demonstrate extensive calcifications and a saccular configuration.

Saccular or fusiform aneurysms of the transverse arch are usually atherosclerotic. Mycotic aneurysms can demonstrate inflammatory changes in the adjacent mediastinal fat and an irregular contour. Descending thoracic aortic aneurysms are most commonly atherosclerotic. A saccular configuration in the proximal aspect of the descending aorta should raise the concern of an aortic transection. A fusiform shape in a descending aneurysm in a younger patient suggests Marfan syndrome, Takayasu arteritis, or other vasculiti as a cause. Aneurysms along the inferior aspect of the proximal aorta may represent a ductus aneurysm. Mycotic aneurysms have a predilection for the distal thoracic aorta in the region of the diaphragm. Posttraumatic aneurysms of the ascending aorta are rarely seen because these patients do not usually survive long enough for a trip to the hospital. These aneurysms instead often involve the descending aorta immediately distal to the origin of the left subclavian artery in the region of the ligamentum arteriosum.

Etiology

Atherosclerosis is the overall most common cause of aortic aneurysms. Others include posttraumatic events, infectious etiologies (mycotic), syphilis, congenital diseases such as Marfan syndrome or Ehlers-Danlos syndrome, and vasculitides such as Takayasu arteritis or Behçet disease.

Epidemiology

As mentioned, different types of aneurysms are more common in patients of specific ages.

Pathogenesis

Atherosclerotic aneurysms are thought to be secondary to a compromised vascular supply to the wall of the vessel with resultant degeneration of the wall. Posttraumatic injuries can be from rapid deceleration motor-vehicle injuries or as a complication of cardiothoracic surgery. Mycotic aneurysms are somewhat of a misnomer, as they are often caused by bacterial infections such as *Staphylococcus*, *Streptococcus*, and *Salmonella*. Syphilitic aneurysms are a long-term sequela of syphilis secondary to infection of the vasa vasorum. Marfan and Ehlers-Danlos cause abnormal tissue formation along the wall of the vessel; this condition is termed *cystic medial necrosis*, and results in pseudoaneurysms.

Diagnostic Evaluation

A CXR is often the first study performed, and it may show abnormal contour of the mediastinum. A CT scan may also be performed and would better delineate the nature of the abnormality. Aortography is used to confirm the findings on CT and can be used in preoperative planning to determine the relationship of the aneurysm to other vessels originating from the aorta.

Radiologic Findings

A normal aortogram should demonstrate the ascending aorta, the aortic arch, and the descending thoracic aorta in their entirety (Figure 10-1). The left anterior oblique projection provides the best visualization of the arch and relevant anatomy. A traumatic aortic pseudoaneurysm typically occurs near the region of the ligamentum arteriosum and demonstrates increased caliber of the vessel compared with the rest of the aorta or a mediastinal hematoma on CT or MRI. It can also be seen on aortography as an abnormal convexity in the contour of the vessel (Figure 10-2). These lesions have

been treated surgically in the past, although placement of endovascular stent grafts has become more frequent.

> ### KEY POINTS
>
> 1. The thoracic aorta is divided into the ascending aorta, the aortic arch, and the descending aorta.
> 2. The most common etiology of thoracic aortic aneurysms is atherosclerosis, although other etiologies include posttraumatic conditions, infectious (mycotic) aneurysms, syphilis, congenital diseases such as Marfan or Ehlers-Danlos, and vasculitides such as Takayasu arteritis or Behçet disease.
> 3. Aortography is useful in preoperative planning to determine the relationship of the aneurysm to other vessels originating from the aorta.

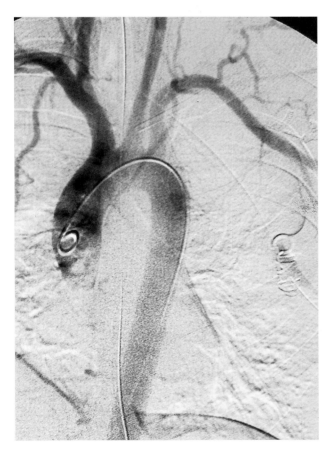

Figure 10-1 • Normal aortic arch in the left anterior oblique (LAO) projection. The aortic arch gives rise to the brachiocephalic artery, the left common carotid and the left subclavian artery.

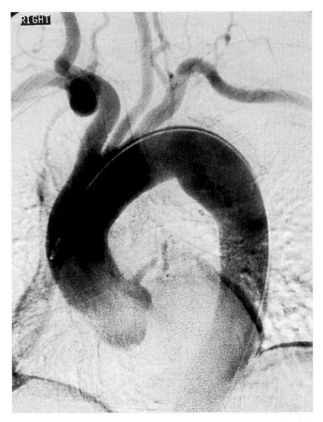

Figure 10-2 • Angiogram of aortic pseudoaneurysm in a patient who was in a motor-vehicle accident. Abnormal contour of the vessel is seen on the inner aspect of the aortic arch distal to the left subclavian artery.
(Courtesy of University of Southern California Medical Center, Los Angeles, CA.)

INFERIOR VENA CAVA FILTER PLACEMENT

Anatomy

The inferior vena cava (IVC) is the largest vein in the body and is situated slightly to the right of the spine. It is formed by the union of the right and left common iliac veins, typically near the level of the L5 vertebral body. The lumbar, renal, right gonadal, and hepatic veins are major tributaries that drain into the IVC during its course through the abdomen. In patients with DVT of the lower extremity, a filter can be placed percutaneously in the IVC to prevent an embolus from traveling superiorly into the pulmonary vasculature.

Etiology and Pathogenesis

The presence of three important factors—venous stasis, endothelial injury, and a hypercoagulable state **(Virchow triad)**—contribute to the formation of venous thrombosis.

Epidemiology

DVT often occurs in patients older than 40 and in people who are immobilized for extended periods (e.g., in hospitalized or bedridden patients).

Clinical Manifestations

History

IVC filters are usually placed in patients with DVT only under certain circumstances, including a contraindication to anticoagulation, a complication from anticoagulation, or failure to prevent PE with anticoagulation. Other relative indications for vena cava filter placement include large, free-floating iliofemoral thrombi and long-term immobilization.

Physical Examination

A DVT in an extremity can manifest as edema, tenderness, or a positive Homan sign (discomfort in the calf muscle with forced dorsiflexion of the foot).

Diagnostic Evaluation

A cavagram is performed before placement of the filter to assess the size of the IVC, to rule out the presence of a thrombus in the IVC or any anatomic anomalies, and to determine the location of the renal veins (Figure 10-3). Many different kinds of filters are available, with properties that make them advantageous in different situations. Certain filters are removable (such as a Gunther Tulip). A Bird's Nest filter can be used in patients with unusually large IVC diameters. Other filters include VenaTech, Simon Nitinol (made of an alloy of nickel and titanium that reforms to a predetermined shape at body temperature), Greenfield (one of the earliest, but with more modern versions), and TrapEase filters (symmetric double-basket shape).

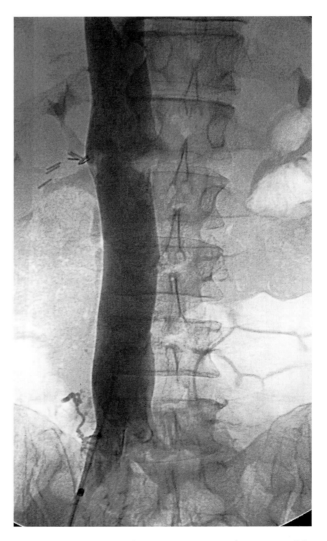

Figure 10-3 • Cavagram demonstrating normal anatomy of the IVC. The apparent filling defects at the L1/L2 disc space represent the inflow of the renal veins.

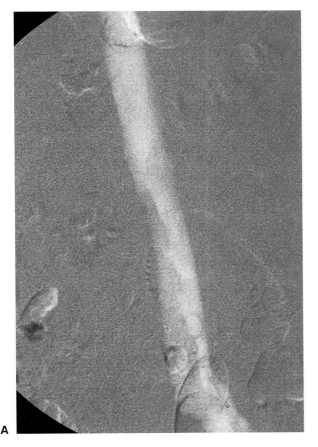

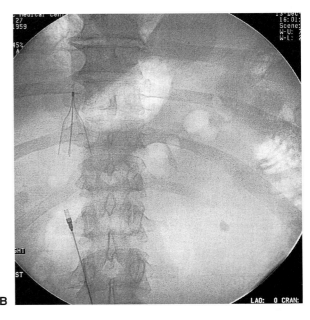

A   **B**

Figure 10-4 • **A:** Cavagram performed with CO_2 as contrast in a patient with renal insufficiency. A long, irregular filling defect is seen along the right lateral edge of the IVC below the level of the renal inflows, consistent with a nonocclusive infrarenal thrombus. **B:** The IVC filter for the same patient was placed at a suprarenal level. Note that this filter is placed much higher than in the previous example, with the proximal tip near the superior endplate of T10.
(Courtesy of University of Southern California Medical Center, Los Angeles, CA.)

Radiologic Findings

After the cavagram is performed, the filter can be placed. The optimal position is just below the level of the renal veins, although if the infrarenal IVC contains a thrombus, it may be necessary to place a suprarenal filter (Figure 10-4). Once the filter is in place, a final film is taken (Figure 10-5 and 10-6).

▓ AORTOILIAC OCCLUSIVE DISEASE

Anatomy

Atherosclerotic disease is a common cause of occlusive disease in the arterial system. The aortoiliac

KEY POINTS

1. IVC filters are placed in patients with DVT and a contraindication to anticoagulation, a complication from anticoagulation, or failure of anticoagulation to prevent PE. Other relative indications for placement include large, free-floating iliofemoral thrombi and long-term immobilization.

2. A cavagram is performed before filter placement to assess the size of the IVC and to evaluate for thrombi within the IVC, anatomic anomalies, and the position of the renal veins.

3. Optimal position of the filter is just below the level of the renal veins.

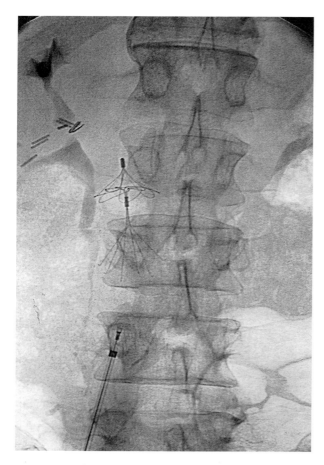

Figure 10-5 · This is an example of a Simon Nitinol filter, which is made of an alloy of nickel and titanium that reforms to a pre-determined shape at body temperature.

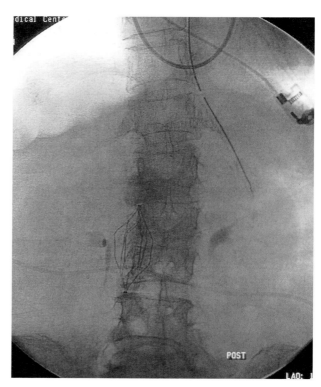

Figure 10-6 · An example of a TrapEase filter. Its design allows it to be easily placed from either a jugular or femoral approach from the same package.
(Courtesy of University of Southern California Medical Center, Los Angeles, CA.)

junction is one of the most common locations for this disease to occur. The aorta typically bifurcates at the L5 or L4–L5 disc space into the right and left common iliac arteries. The common iliac artery then bifurcates into the external iliac and internal iliac arteries. The external iliac artery continues to the common femoral artery to supply the lower extremities, although it gives off the circumflex iliac and inferior epigastric branches in the pelvis. The internal iliac artery supplies the organs of the pelvis (see Figure 10-7). The internal iliac artery has highly variable anatomy, but typically it is divided into posterior and anterior divisions. The branches of the posterior division are the iliolumbar, superior gluteal, and lateral sacral arteries. The anterior division includes the inferior gluteal, obturator, middle rectal, internal pudendal, uterine (in females), and vesicle branches.

Etiology

This disorder is caused by plaque formation that develops over many years and is related to a number of risk factors, including elevated cholesterol levels, hypertension, cigarette smoking, diabetes, and several others.

Epidemiology

Because this disease develops gradually, it is typically diagnosed in older patients who have the risk factors described in the preceding section.

Pathogenesis

Atherosclerosis is thought to arise as a result of arterial injury. An inflammatory response to endothelial injury will cause lipid accumulation in the arterial wall, which then stimulates platelet aggregation and clot formation.

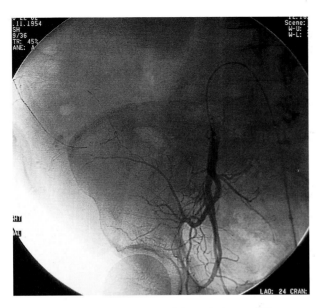

Figure 10-7 · Selective injection of the right internal iliac artery. There is good visualization of the normal pelvic arterial branches (see text).
(Courtesy of University of Southern California Medical Center, Los Angeles, CA.)

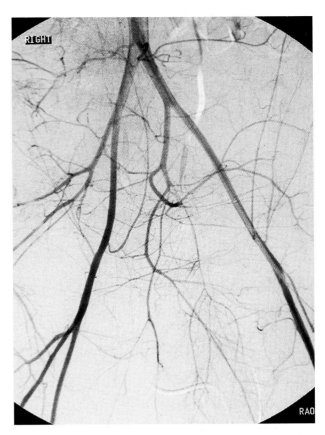

Figure 10-8 · Normal pelvic angiography with catheter positioned in the distal aorta, demonstrating bilateral iliac arteries and their branches.

Clinical Manifestations

History

Patients may present with claudication, thigh and buttock pain, impotence, or vascular compromise of the lower extremity. The triad of buttock claudication, decreased femoral pulses, and impotence is described as **Leriche syndrome.** However, as many as half of patients with this disease may be asymptomatic.

Physical Examination

Patients can demonstrate deceased peripheral pulses and decreased ankle-brachial indices (ABIs).

Diagnostic Evaluation

If nonmedical therapies such as angioplasty, stent placement, or surgery are being considered, ultrasound, MRA, or conventional angiography may be performed.

Radiologic Findings

Normal abdominal and pelvic angiography demonstrates relatively straight vessels with smooth contour (Figure 10-8). In patients with atherosclerotic disease, these vessels can demonstrate narrowing, tortu-

osity, irregular contours, calcifications, focal dilatations, and occlusion of segments (Figure 10-9). These lesions can be treated by a number of methods. Percutaneous transluminal angioplasty (PTA) or intraluminal stent placement can be performed by an interventional radiologist. Several surgical options also exist to treat this disease.

KEY POINTS

1. The aortoiliac junction is a common site of involvement for atherosclerotic disease.
2. The involved vessels demonstrate narrowing, tortuosity, irregular contours, calcifications, focal dilatations, and occlusion of segments.
3. Treatment options include PTA, intraluminal stent placement, and axillofemoral bypass.

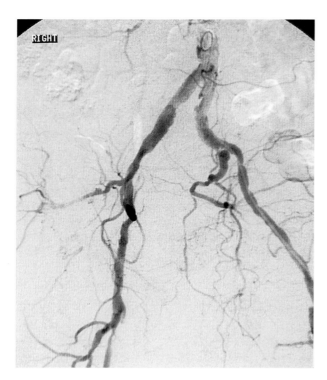

Figure 10-9 • Pelvic angiogram in a patient with tortuous, irregular vessels, consistent with aortoiliac atherosclerotic disease.

PERIPHERAL VASCULAR DISEASE

Anatomy

The common femoral artery is a direct extension of the external iliac artery, beginning at the inguinal ligament. Just distal to the inferior aspect of the femoral head, the femoral artery branches into the profunda femoris and the superficial femoral arteries (see Figure 10-10). The profunda femoris artery (PFA) arises from the posterolateral aspect of the artery and travels medial to the femur and deep to the superficial femoral artery (SFA), giving off several muscular branches. The SFA runs underneath the sartorius muscle medial and anterior to the PFA and passes through the adductor canal, after which it becomes the popliteal artery.

The popliteal artery supplies the knee via superior and inferior (both medial and lateral) and middle geniculate branches. The popliteal artery then divides into the anterior tibial artery (arising laterally) and the tibioperoneal trunk. The tibioperoneal trunk runs for a short distance before dividing into the posterior tibial (arising medially) and the peroneal arteries (see Figure 10-11).

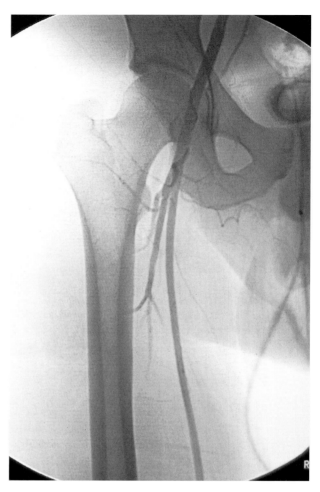

Figure 10-10 • Normal angiogram of the arteries of the right proximal thigh, including the common femoral artery, profunda femoris artery (PFA), and the superficial femoral artery (SFA). Note the medial position of the SFA in relation to the PFA. (Courtesy of University of Southern California Medical Center, Los Angeles, CA.)

Etiology

As in aortoiliac occlusive disease, atherosclerotic disease is the most common causative agent in chronic peripheral vascular occlusion. Other less common causes include Burger disease (thromboangiitis obliterans), vasculitis, popliteal entrapment syndrome, adventitial cystic disease, radiation, trauma, and chronic emboli.

Epidemiology

This disease is actually quite prevalent, affecting 20% of people older than 70 years of age. However, fewer than half of people with the disease are symptomatic.

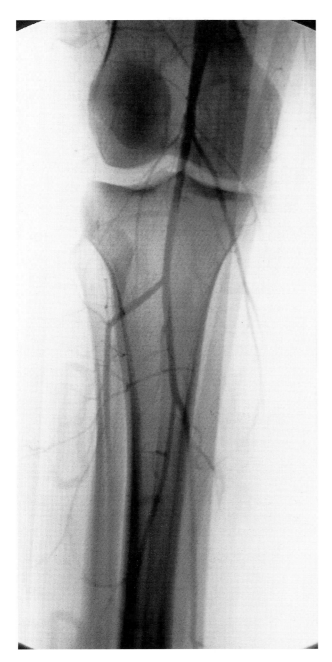

Figure 10-11 • Normal angiogram of the arteries around the knee. The popliteal artery gives off the anterior tibial artery just below the knee; note its lateral position, adjacent to the fibula. The tibioperoneal trunk then travels for a short distance before branching into the posterior tibial (medially located) and the peroneal arteries.
(Courtesy of University of Southern California Medical Center, Los Angeles, CA.)

Pathogenesis

The pathogenesis of peripheral vascular disease is also related to the atherosclerotic process, similar to aortoiliac occlusive disease.

Clinical Manifestations

History

Claudication is the first symptom to develop; patients with more severe disease may develop rest pain, skin changes (atrophy, scaling, hair loss), ulceration, and tissue necrosis. Atherosclerotic peripheral vascular disease correlates strongly with systemic atherosclerotic vascular disease. Patients with severe symptomatic peripheral vascular disease have a mortality rate from cardiovascular causes that is several times higher than that of control groups.

Physical Examination

Because this disease most often shares the same etiology as aortoiliac occlusive disease, deceased peripheral pulses and decreased ABIs can also be seen.

Diagnostic Evaluation

Again, as with aortoiliac occlusive disease, if nonmedical therapies such as angioplasty, stent placement, or surgery are being considered, ultrasound, MRA, or conventional angiography may be performed.

Radiologic Findings

Peripheral vascular disease will demonstrate stenosis or occlusion of major vessels (Figure 10-12). CT angiography and MRA are also useful in evaluating this disease. If the disease is severe and extensive, surgical bypass remains the best option. Percutaneous intervention is best suited for lesions that are focal and less than 5 cm long. PTA, stents, stent-grafts, and thrombolysis have all been used successfully in some capacity.

KEY POINTS

1. As with aortoiliac occlusive disease, atherosclerosis is the most common cause of peripheral vascular disease.
2. Claudiation is usually a patient's first symptom. More severe disease may result in rest pain, skin changes, ulceration, or tissue necrosis.
3. Percutaneous intervention is best suited for focal lesions that are less than 5 cm long.

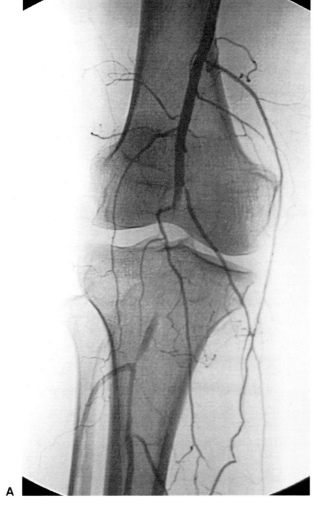

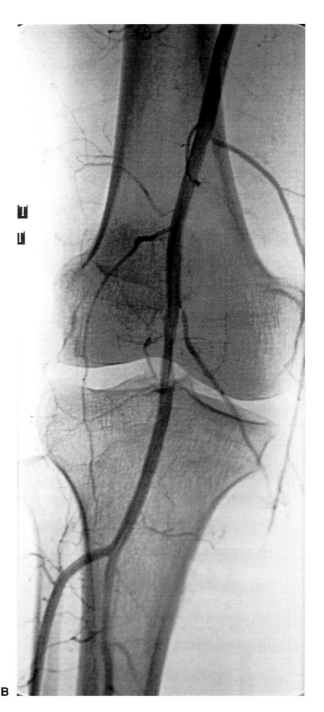

A

B

A: Angiogram of the right lower extremity in a patient with peripheral vascular disease evidenced by a foot ulcer. The popliteal artery demonstrates an occlusion at the level of the knee joint. **B:** Angiogram of the patient in (A) after percutaneous transluminal angioplasty. The popliteal artery is now widely patent.
(Courtesy of University of Southern California Medical Center, Los Angeles, CA.)

■ GASTROINTESTINAL HEMORRHAGE

Anatomy

GI hemorrhage is usually classified as either upper or lower, depending on whether the source is proximal or distal to the ligament of Treitz. Upper GI hemorrhage is typically from vessels originating from the celiac axis, including the right and left gastric arteries and the gastroduodenal artery. Lower GI hemorrhage can occur from branches of both the superior (supplying the small bowel and right colon) and the inferior mesenteric (supplying the left colon sigmoid and rectum) arteries.

Etiology and Pathogenesis

Causes for upper GI hemorrhage include varices, Mallory-Weiss tears, peptic ulcers, gastritis, angiodysplasia, hemobilia, iatrogenic and aortoenteric fistulas, and tumors. Common causes of lower GI hemorrhage include diverticular disease, angiodysplasia, cancer, hemorrhoids, Meckel diverticulum, inflammatory bowel disease, radiation colitis, and ischemic bowel. GI hemorrhage is several times more common from the upper GI tract and occurs most commonly from ulcers or gastritis. The most common source of lower GI bleeding is from the colon; diverticulosis and angiodysplasia are the most common causes.

Clinical Manifestations

History

Patients typically present with hematemesis in the case of upper GI hemorrhage or with melena or hematochezia in lower GI hemorrhage. Acute hemorrhage usually resolves spontaneously (in up to 85% of patients). Patients who are unresponsive to supportive measures undergo endoscopic evaluation. Endoscopy is more sensitive in detecting the source of upper than lower GI bleeds. In the event the patient continues to hemorrhage and a source cannot be found, angiography can be performed. Angiograms demonstrate a source of bleeding in only about half of patients.

Physical Examination

Patients with lower GI bleeding may demonstrate melena, hematochezia, or hemodynamic instability. Upper GI bleeding can present with hematemesis, coffee-ground emesis or coffee grounds seen in nasogastric lavage, melena, or even hematochezia if the rate of bleeding is high; hemodynamic instability is also seen.

Diagnostic Evaluation

Endoscopy remains the most valuable method of both identifying and treating both upper and lower GI hemorrhage. However, in some cases the site of hemorrhage is not seen on endoscopy. In these cases, radionuclide scintigraphy has been very sensitive in identifying hemorrhage, although the site is sometimes difficult to determine. Angiography and embolization have been shown to be very effective in these patients.

Radiologic Findings

Hemorrhage is identified on angiography as a small collection of contrast outside of the normal course of the vessel within the bowel lumen (Figure 10-13a). The contrast should persist beyond the arterial phase and will change with time. Once the source of bleeding is identified, a smaller catheter can be positioned closer to the bleeding vessel if desired. Vasopressin (a smooth-muscle constrictor), embolization coils, embolization glue, or other occlusive materials such as gelfoam or large particles can be administered through the catheter directly into the vessel to stop the hemorrhage (Figure 10-13b). Embolization can be performed if the exact site of bleeding is identified; the most distal vessel demonstrating the hemorrhage should always be chosen.

KEY POINTS

1. Angiography can be performed if a source for GI hemorrhage cannot be identified by endoscopy.
2. Once a source is identified, various embolic materials or vasopressin can be administered directly into the vessel to stop the bleeding.

■ PERCUTANEOUS NEPHROSTOMY TUBE

Anatomy

The kidneys are located in the retroperitoneum at the level of T12 to L3. The right kidney is a few centimeters lower than the left, presumably because of the larger size of the right lobe of the liver. The superior aspects of the kidneys are covered by the lower ribs, and the kidneys are oriented obliquely so that

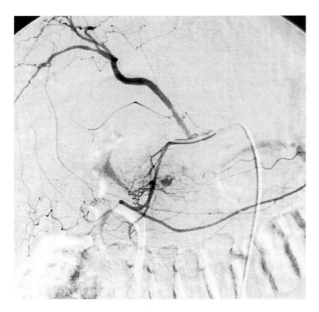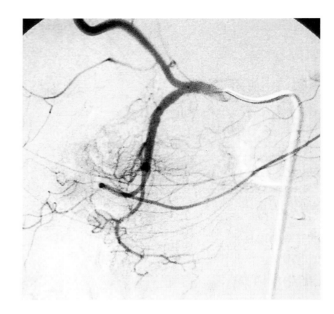

Figure 10-13 • **A:** Angiogram of the common hepatic artery, with an irregular collection of extraluminal contrast medial to the gastroduodenal artery in this patient with a GI bleed. **B:** After embolization of the bleeding vessel, the extraluminal spill of contrast is no longer seen.

the location of the inferior poles is more anterior than that of the superior poles. These are important facts to remember because they affect the percutaneous approach to these organs, which is done posteriorly with the patient lying prone.

Etiology/Pathogenesis

Hydronephrosis is dilatation of the renal collecting system, usually from an obstruction of a ureter, the bladder, or the urethra. A drainage catheter can be placed percutaneously into the collecting system to relieve such obstructions. Obstruction of the renal collecting system can occur from the presence of a stone; a tumor in the ureter, bladder, or adjacent organs such as the colon, prostate, cervix or uterus; idiopathic retroperitoneal fibrosis; enlarged lymph nodes; or as a sequela of prior surgery.

Epidemiology

Hydronephrosis from benign prostatic hypertrophy or prostate cancer is more common in older men. In women, pregnancy and cervical cancer are more common causes. In younger adults, kidney stones are the most common cause, and in children ureteropelvic junction obstructions and vesicoureteral reflux are common causes.

Clinical Manifestations

History

Hydronephrosis may present with pain, nausea, vomiting, decreased urine output, or it may be asymptomatic.

Physical Examination

Lower-extremity edema, flank tenderness, or a palpable flank mass can be seen on physical examination, depending on the etiology and severity of the hydronephrosis.

Diagnostic Evaluation

Ultrasound is a quick and simple method of identifying hydronephrosis. Plain films can demonstrate calcifications if they are present. CT is sensitive in identifying the presence as well as the cause of hydronephrosis. Radionuclide studies can demonstrate whether a hydronephrotic kidney is functioning properly.

Radiologic Findings

Normal calyces and ureters, shown in the normal intravenous pyelogram, demonstrate smooth contours without dilatation of the renal calyces, pelves, and

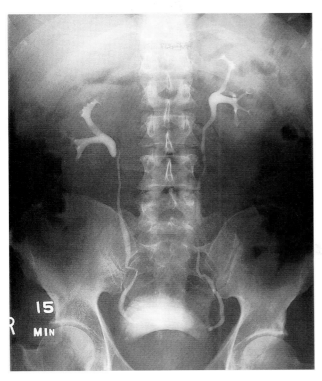

Figure 10-14 • Normal intravenous pyelogram (IVP). Note the smooth, regular contours of the renal calyces, pelvis, and ureters. (Courtesy of University of Southern California Medical Center, Los Angeles, CA.)

KEY POINTS

1. Obstruction of the renal collecting system can occur from the presence of a stone; a tumor in the ureter, bladder, or adjacent organs such as the colon, prostate, cervix, or uterus; retroperitoneal fibrosis; enlarged lymph nodes; or as a sequela of prior surgery.
2. Percutaneous nephrostomy catheters can be placed for relief of urinary obstruction, urinary diversion, or for access for further diagnostic or interventional procedures.

ABSCESS DRAINAGE

Fluid collections can occur in many parts of the body, often from infection. Complicated pleural effusions and infected intra-abdominal fluid collections are often drained under CT or ultrasound guidance, with or without the placement of an indwelling percutaneous catheter with a coiled tip (several different types of catheters are available). Percutaneous drainage has largely replaced surgical intervention as

ureters (Figure 10-14). Dilated calyces are readily identified under ultrasound. Nephrostomy catheters are usually placed posteriorly because the kidneys lie in the retroperitoneal space. Placement of catheters directly into the renal pelvis should be avoided because of their proximity to the main renal vessels; it is preferable to place the catheter through a renal calyx into the renal pelvis. Placement into a posterior calyx produces less of an angle for the entry of catheters than does placement into an anterior calyx.

With the patient in prone position, a needle is typically advanced under ultrasound guidance into a posterior calyx. A small amount of contrast is then injected under fluoroscopy to confirm its location within the calyx. This should also demonstrate dilatation of the calyces in a patient with hydronephrosis. Once the position is confirmed, a catheter can be placed for urinary drainage (Figure 10-15). Nephrostomy tubes can also be placed for urinary diversion to allow distal leaks to heal and for access to the collecting system for diagnostic and interventional procedures.

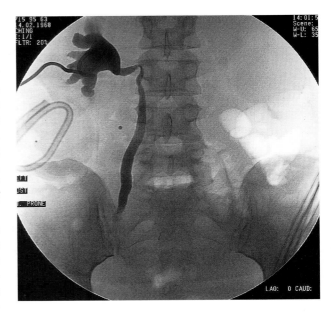

Figure 10-15 • This patient has cervical cancer causing obstruction of the left ureter in the pelvis. A nephostomy tube was placed in the left renal pelvis via a lower pole calyx. Note that because the patient is lying prone for this procedure, the left side of the patient appears on the left side of the image. (Courtesy of University of Southern California Medical Center, Los Angeles, CA.)

an initial treatment for these collections. The preferred course of the catheter is typically the one with the shortest distance from the skin, avoiding any major vascular or visceral structures.

Etiology

Intra-abdominal fluid collections can result from a number of causes, including infection after a prior surgery, perforation of a visceral organ, pyogenic liver abscess, biloma, pancreatic pseudocyst or abscess, urinoma, perinephric abscess, or tubo-ovarian abscesses. Pleural fluid can be serous, (hydrothorax), blood (hemothorax), lipid (chylothorax), and pus (pyothorax or empyema).

Diagnostic Evaluation

The fluid collection must be clearly identified to be treated. CT or ultrasound can show the location of the collection and its relationship to adjacent structures and demonstrate a window for a catheter or needle to be placed.

Radiologic Findings

An abscess on CT is lower in attenuation than the surrounding soft tissues, but it is higher than fat. It

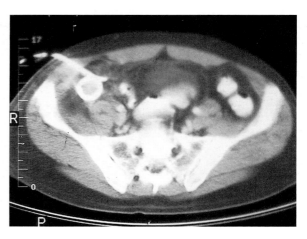

Figure 10-17 • A percutaneous pigtail drainage catheter has been placed using CT guidance in the abscess with the amount of fluid much smaller or gone altogether.
(Courtesy of University of Southern California Medical Center, Los Angeles, CA.)

will often have a thick, enhancing rim, with increased density (stranding) of the adjacent fat (Figure 10-16). A catheter can be placed using CT periodically to take images and to evaluate the exact position of the catheter. Once in place, a final image is obtained to document the location of the catheter within the fluid collection (Figure 10-17).

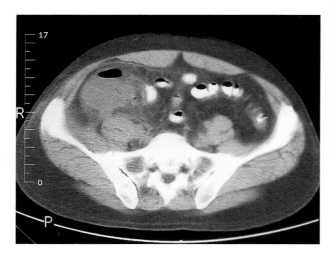

Figure 10-16 • Axial CT of the pelvis with oral contrast demonstrates a large fluid collection anterior to the right psoas muscle with associated gas and adjacent inflammatory changes in this patient, who has a right lower quadrant intra-abdominal abscess.
(Courtesy of University of Southern California Medical Center, Los Angeles, CA.)

KEY POINTS

1. CT or ultrasound can be used to guide percutaneous placement of catheters to drain a fluid collection or abscess in nearly any part of the body.
2. An abscess on CT is lower in attenuation than the surrounding soft tissues, but it is higher than fat. It will often have a thick, enhancing rim with increased density (stranding) of the adjacent fat.

Nuclear Medicine

Nuclear medicine uses small amounts of radioactive substances administered to patients and detects the radiation emitted from inside the body to produce images (scintigrams) of organs based on physiology rather than on anatomy. Some studies are obtained over time for a functional evaluation. The chemical compounds are radiopharmaceuticals (tracers) with physiologic properties. The radioactive substances attached to them are radionuclides that emit gamma radiation or beta radiation. The most current radionuclides used in nuclear medicine and their physical properties are summarized in Table 11-1. The radiation emitted from inside the body is detected by gamma cameras. The gamma cameras include a collimator, a sodium iodide (NaI) crystal, an array of photomultiplier tubes, and an electronic circuitry attached to a computer that generates images based on the radiation detected from the patient (Figure 11-1). The images can be planar (from a single gamma camera in fixed relation to the patient) or spatially reconstructed from one, two, or three gamma camera detectors around the patient (single-photon emission computed tomography, or SPECT).

The radiation emitted inside the body allows attempts at curative targeted therapy in thyroid cancer (iodine-131, or ^{131}I) and certain lymphomas (radiolabelled antibodies) or symptom palliation in bone metastases (strontium-89, or ^{89}Sr).

■ SKELETAL

Nuclear medicine skeletal studies are useful in the early detection of bone lesions of various etiologies and to survey the entire skeleton. The radiopharmaceuticals currently used are diphosphonates that accumulate in bone lesions, depending on the local osteoblastic activity and the blood flow. They are labeled with technetium-99m (^{99m}Tc).

Indications

Bone scans are used to detect osseous metastasis (prostate cancer, breast cancer), Paget disease, stress fractures, and skeletal changes associated with metabolic processes (osteomalacia, renal osteodystrophy).

■ TABLE 11-1

Physical Properties of Most Commonly Used Radionuclides in Clinical Nuclear Medicine

Radionuclide	Physical Half-Life	Principal Photon Energy (keV)
Technetium (Tc)-99m	6 hr	140
Iodine (I)-131	8 days	364
Iodine (I)-123	13.2 hr	159
Gallium (Ga)-67	78.3 hr	93, 185, 300, 395
Thallium (Tl)-201	73.1 hr	69–83, 135
Indium (In)-111	2.8 days	171, 245
Xenon (Xe)-133	5.2 days	81

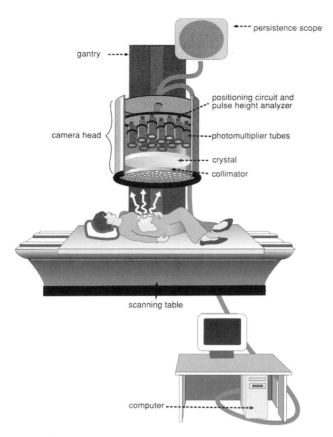

Figure 11-1 • Components of a standard gamma camera.
(Reprinted with permission from Powsner, R. *Essentials of Nuclear Medicine Physics,* Figure 6.1, p. 79, Malden, MA: Blackwell Publishing, 1998.)

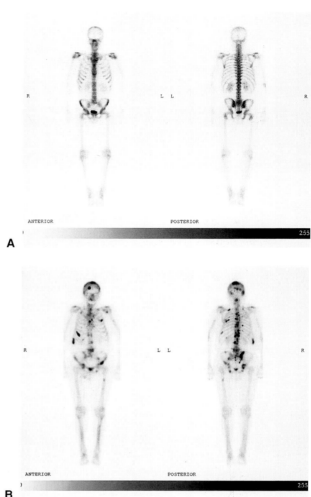

Figure 11-2 • A: Normal bone scan B: Multiple bone metastases in a patient with prostate cancer.
(Courtesy of University of Southern California Medical Center, Los Angeles, CA.)

In instances of suspected child abuse in which plain x-ray films fail to identify fractures, bone scans may provide additional diagnostic data.

A three-phase bone scan adds images of arterial blood flow and blood pool (tracer at equilibrium in soft tissue) to a bone scan and is useful for detecting infection and reflex sympathetic dystrophy.

Normal Scintigraphy

Normal uptake is present in bones (it should be uniform and symmetric), soft tissues throughout the body (creating background activity), epiphyses (in pediatric patients), and breasts (which should be symmetric). The tracer has renal clearance, and the kidneys and urinary bladder are normally visualized (Figure 11-2A). The images obtained are nonspecific and very often should be interpreted in the clinical context and, if needed, correlated with anatomic imaging.

Abnormal Findings

Multiple foci of randomly distributed hypermetabolic lesions are consistent with bone metastases in cancer patients (Figure 11-2B), but even a single abnormal focus of radiotracer uptake can represent primary bone tumor (Figure 11-3) or metastasis. Some bone metastases appear as photopenic areas (renal cancer). Uniformly increased radiotracer accumulation in a vertebral body in an elderly person can represent compression fracture. Images should be correlated with anatomic studies.

Increased radiotracer localization in all three phases of a bone scan is suggestive of osteomyelitis.

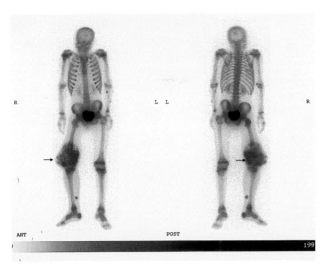

Figure 11-3 • Bone scan in a patient with right distal femur osteosarcoma *(arrows)*.
(Courtesy of University of Southern California Medical Center, Los Angeles, CA.)

KEY POINTS

1. Bone imaging depends on the local osteoblastic activity and the blood flow.
2. Images should be interpreted in the clinical context and with anatomic correlation.

■ PULMONARY

Evaluation of patients with suspected PE is the single most important use of pulmonary nuclear medicine. V/Q are becoming second-line diagnostic tools in recent years as a result of the widely accepted and available computed tomography pulmonary angiography (CTPA). The V/Q study consists of two phases: evaluation of ventilation after administration of a radioactive gas (usually xenon-133, or ^{133}Xe) and evaluation of pulmonary perfusion after intravenous injection of ^{99m}Tc macroaggregated albumin (MAA) (Figure 11-4A). The study is evaluated in conjunction with a chest x-ray because the results may be equivocal in patients with pre-existing lung disease. The results are expressed as probability (high, intermediate, low), which should be interpreted in the context of clinical suspicion and pretest probability for a PE. The diagnostic criteria are derived from the Prospective Investigation of Pulmonary Embolism Diagnosis (PIOPED) study.

Indications

V/Q scans remain valuable in evaluation for PE of pediatric and pregnant patients, when a lower radiation exposure is warranted, or when CTPA cannot be performed (as with renal failure, contrast allergy). V/Q studies are useful in the follow-up of patients

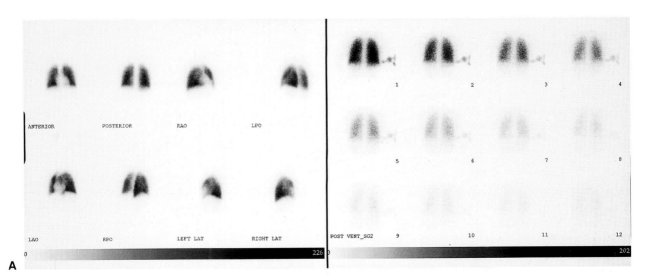

Figure 11-4 • **A:** Normal V/Q scan. **B:** Normal ventilation but multiple perfusion defects in a study interpreted as high probability for pulmonary embolism.
(Courtesy of University of Southern California Medical Center, Los Angeles, CA.)

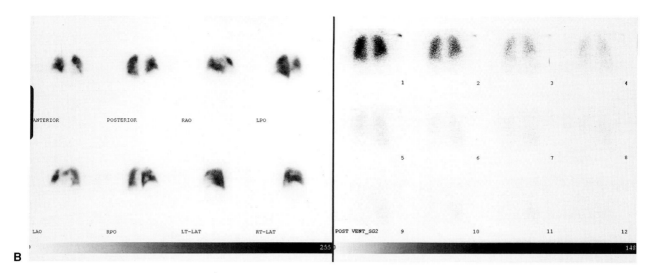

B

Figure 11-4 • continued

with chronic PE and as part of the evaluation of lung function before surgery. Quantitative scans provide relative estimations of pulmonary function and can be used both before and after lung transplantation.

Abnormal Findings

The classic PE appearance on a V/Q scan is segmental (wedge shaped), pleural-based perfusion defects, not matched by ventilation defects (Figure 11-4B).

KEY POINTS

1. V/Q scans remain valuable diagnostic tools in pediatric and pregnant patients and in patients with renal failure or contrast allergy.
2. Interpretation is based on the PIOPED criteria, and results are expressed as probabilities.

▉ CARDIOVASCULAR

Current protocols use SPECT imaging, with planar studies reserved for special instances (e.g., in obese patients). The SPECT study includes a rest acquisition (usually with thallium-201) and a poststress acquisition (using ^{99m}Tc tracers). Several protocols regarding the sequencing of the acquisitions are available. The stress can be treadmill exercise or pharmacologic (dipyridamole, adenosine, or dobutamine). Coupling the poststress images with an electrocardiogram (ECG) tracing is called **gating,** and it allows the computer to generate estimations of cardiac function (ejection fraction, end diastolic volume) and to create images of wall motion.

Cardiac nuclear medicine can be used for evaluation of the functional status of the heart. Red blood cells tagged with ^{99m}Tc show the cardiac blood-pool images over time, which allows a cinematic display of the left ventricular motion and an exact estimation of the ejection fraction. The study is called multiple-gated angiography (MUGA).

Indications

The diagnosis of coronary artery disease (CAD), risk stratification after myocardial infarction (MI), preoperative evaluation, and assessment of viable myocardium versus scar are the main indications for myocardial perfusion scintigraphy. MUGA scans can evaluate the cardiac function before and after potentially cardiotoxic chemotherapy (i.e., doxorubicin).

Normal Scintigraphy

Normal scintigraphy shows uniform distribution of the radiotracer in the left ventricular myocardium on both the stress and resting images (Figure 11-5A). Normal MUGA reveals normal left ventricular wall motion and an ejection fraction greater than 50%.

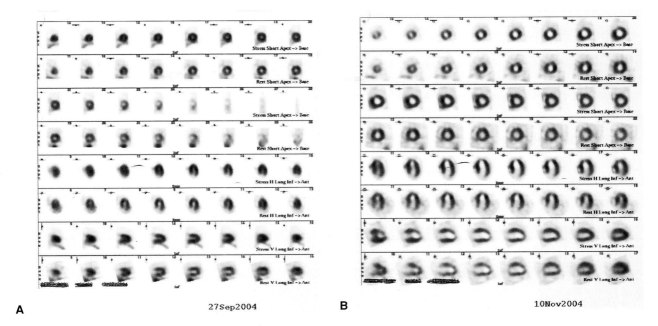

Figure 11-5 • A: Normal cardiac scintigraphy demonstrating uniform radiotracer distribution in the left ventricular myocardium. **B:** Abnormal cardiac stress study showing ischemia of the apicoseptal wall of the left ventricle *(arrows)*. (Courtesy of University of Southern California Medical Center, Los Angeles, CA.)

Abnormal Findings

Ischemic areas show decreased uptake of radiotracer on the stress images compared with the rest images (reversible defect) (Figure 11-5B). Areas of MI appear as perfusion defects on both images (fixed defect). Artifacts can occur and are secondary to motion or soft-tissue attenuation from breast (anterior wall) or diaphragm (inferior wall). Multivessel CAD produces global ischemia and can render a study normal because there are no areas of diminished perfusion relative to the rest of the myocardium. This is called **balanced ischemia.** Wall-motion abnormalities and a decreased ejection fraction should be noted on a MUGA scan.

KEY POINTS

1. Myocardial perfusion scintigraphy is a major diagnostic and prognostic tool in the evaluation of cardiac pathology.
2. MUGA is the most accurate procedure in calculating left ventricular ejection fraction.

▇ HEPATOBILIARY

The main application of nuclear medicine in hepatobiliary imaging is currently cholescintigraphy using ^{99m}Tc hepatoiminodiacetic acid analogues (HIDA scans). HIDA scintigraphy can detect hepatic and biliary tract pathology because the tracer is cleared by the liver from the blood pool, excreted into the biliary tree, accumulated in the GB, and released in the bowel. The patient must fast 4 hours before the study but no longer than 24 hours (an already-filled GB will not be visualized).

^{99m}Tc sulphur colloid is taken up by the reticuloendothelial system and can be used to image the liver and spleen when CT cannot be performed (e.g., with contrast allergy, renal failure).

Indications

Indications to perform a HIDA scan are suspicion of acute cholecystitis, acalculous cholecystitis, biliary atresia, biliary leak following cholecystectomy or liver transplant, and evaluation of graft functionality after liver transplant.

^{99m}Tc sulphur colloid scintigraphy is indicated for detection of accessory splenic tissue post splenectomy.

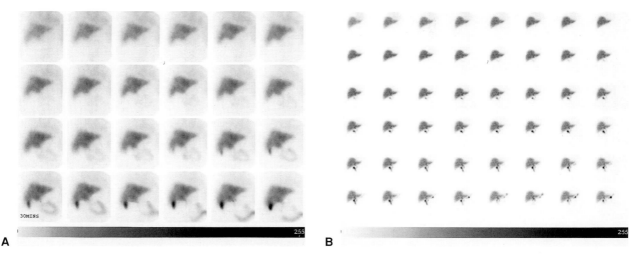

Figure 11-6 • A: Normal HIDA scan, with gallbladder seen at less than 30 minutes *(arrow).* **B:** Abnormal HIDA scintigraphy without visualization of gallbladder up to 1 hour, demonstrating radiotracer in the bowel *(arrow).* The gallbladder was not visualized at 4 hours (not shown), suggesting acute cholecystitis.
(Courtesy of University of Southern California Medical Center, Los Angeles, CA.)

Normal Scintigraphy

Normal HIDA scans should demonstrate prompt radiotracer clearance from the blood pool, visualization of biliary tree by 20 minutes, and visualization of gallbladder and bowel by 60 minutes. The activity in the liver should decrease over time, with little remaining at 1 hour (Figure 11-6A).

Abnormal Findings

Failure to visualize the gallbladder at 1 hour and after morphine administration or on delayed images (4 hours) is consistent with acute cholecystitis (Figure 11-6B). The presence of radiotracer in the blood pool longer than 10 to 15 minutes after injection suggests poor hepatocellular function; absence of visualization of the biliary tree can be secondary to cholelithiasis.

KEY POINTS

1. Patients must fast 4 hours before the study, but no more than 24 hours, to avoid false-positive results on HIDA scans
2. The diagnosis of acute cholecystitis should be confirmed with morphine administration or delayed images.

■ GASTROINTESTINAL

Upper GI hemorrhage can be confirmed with flexible fiberoptic endoscopy, but identification of the site of lower GI bleeding can be difficult. The bleeding scan can help in this instance. It uses ^{99m}Tc-labeled red blood cells.

Radionuclide gastric emptying studies are widely used in evaluating gastric motility. A meal consisting of a scrambled-egg sandwich labeled with ^{99m}Tc sulphur colloid is used in most nuclear medicine departments. Imaging of the stomach is obtained by up to 120 minutes. The processed data allow calculation of the gastric half emptying time ($t\frac{1}{2}$).

^{99m}Tc pertechnetate is secreted by the gastric mucosa and makes this radiotracer valuable in the diagnosis of ectopic gastric mucosa, like Meckel diverticulum.

Indications

Indications include suspicion of GI bleeding in the presence of negative endoscopy or angiography. The GI bleeding scan is able to detect bleeds at rates of 0.5 mL per minute, whereas angiography can detect rates greater than 1 mL per minute.

The gastric emptying scan is indicated to evaluate gastroparesis, dumping syndrome, and any other gastric motility abnormalities.

The Meckel scan is considered the standard method for initial diagnosis of Meckel diverticulum.

Normal Scintigraphy

Normal GI bleed scan shows the radiotracer present in the blood pool, allowing visualization of the heart and the major vessels. Prompt gastric emptying and an absence of radiotracer in the stomach at the end of the study characterize a normal gastric emptying scintigraphy. Normal values for the $t\frac{1}{2}$ of gastric emptying are up to 90 minutes.

Radiotracer uptake should not be seen outside the expected location of the stomach on a negative Meckel scintigraphy.

Abnormal Findings

For a GI bleed study to be positive, the extravascular activity should be in the bowel's lumen, increase over time, and move through the GI tract (Figure 11-7). It is important to provide information about the location of the bleed in a general region (e.g., small bowel, hepatic flexure, transverse colon, splenic flexure, rectosigmoid), guiding the angiographer as to the vessel in which contrast is to be injected.

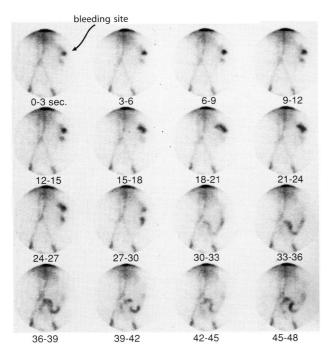

Figure 11-7 • Positive GI bleeding scan.
(Reprinted with permission from Powsner R. *Essentials of Nuclear Medicine Physics*, Figure 6.28, p. 104, Malden, MA: Blackwell Publishing, 1998.)

Rapid gastric emptying is seen postoperatively (e.g., with pyloroplasty or hemigastrectomy) and in gastrinoma and hyperthyroidism. The most common cause of delayed emptying is diabetic gastroparesis. Gastroesophageal reflux can be visualized throughout the study, if it is present.

The Meckel diverticulum appears on a positive scan as a focal area of increased intra-abdominal activity, most frequently in the right lower quadrant.

KEY POINTS

1. The GI bleeding scan is more sensitive than angiography, but the intermittent character of bleeding should be considered in a negative study.
2. The Meckel scan is the gold standard for diagnosing Meckel diverticulum.

■ GENITOURINARY

Nuclear medicine's main renal procedures include dynamic (functional) studies and cortical scans. The most commonly used radiotracers are ^{99m}Tc DTPA and ^{99m}Tc MAG3 for functional studies and ^{99m}Tc DMSA for cortical studies.

^{99m}Tc DTPA is cleared by glomerular filtration and can be used for calculation of the glomerular filtration rate (GFR). ^{99m}Tc MAG3 is cleared by tubular excretion. The study is helpful in describing the renal blood flow, the extraction of the tracer by the kidneys, and its excretion into the collecting system, thus characterizing the renal function and the patency of the urinary tract.

^{99m}Tc DMSA binds to sulfhydryl groups in the renal cortex, and only a small percentage of the radiotracer is cleared by the kidneys, thus allowing cortical visualization.

Radionuclide cystography is used to diagnose vesicoureteral reflux.

Indications

Indications for ^{99m}Tc DTPA/^{99m}Tc MAG3 scans are evaluation of suspected nonfunctional or hypofunctional kidneys, obstruction of urinary tract, and poor function or suspected urine leak after kidney transplantation.

^{99m}Tc DMSA scan is used in suspected pyelonephritis-induced scarring, which is evidenced by renal cortex defects. SPECT imaging allows detection of small defects and makes the study more sensitive than cross-sectional imaging (e.g., ultrasound, CT).

Radionuclide cystography is considered the imaging modality of choice for the evaluation and follow-up of children with urinary tract infections and reflux.

Normal Scintigraphy

Normal ^{99m}Tc DTPA/^{99m}Tc MAG3 scans indicate symmetric, prompt bilateral blood flow; prompt uptake of the radiotracer by the cortex; and rapid bilateral clearance from the cortex, with excretion into the collecting system and urinary bladder. Furosemide (Lasix) can be administered intravenously in cases where obstruction is suspected, with clearance of the tracer more than 20 minutes after injection, suggesting obstruction.

Uniform, homogeneous cortical appearance should be seen on a ^{99m}Tc DMSA scan.

Normal radionuclide cystography should show no activity in the areas corresponding to the ureters or kidneys.

Abnormal Findings

Abnormal ^{99m}Tc DTPA/^{99m}Tc MAG3 scans are suggested by asymmetric renal blood flow; asymmetric or delayed radiotracer extraction and excretion; and tracer stasis in the collecting system.

Renal cortex surface defects on a ^{99m}Tc MAG3 scan are suggestive of postinfection scarring.

Abnormal findings on a radionuclide cystography include any reflux detected as activity above the bladder.

KEY POINTS

1. Renal scintigraphy allows evaluation of renal function in both native and transplanted kidneys.
2. Radionuclide cystography is the imaging modality of choice for the evaluation and follow-up of children with urinary tract infections and reflux.

■ INFECTION

The main agents used for identification of infection are indium-111 (^{111}In)-labeled WBCs, gallium citrate 67 (^{67}Ga), and ^{99m}Tc HMPAO-labeled WBCs.

Indications

Indications are specific and are determined for each agent, including fever of unknown origin, osteomyelitis, intra-abdominal infection, inflammatory bowel disease, and surgical prosthetic graft infection.

Normal Scintigraphy

Normal infection scans with the already-described agents should demonstrate only the physiologic distribution of the radiotracer.

Abnormal Findings

Any activity outside the physiologic radiotracer distribution suggests infection in the corresponding clinical context.

KEY POINTS

1. Each infection seeking agent has specific indications that should be followed in clinical practice.

■ ONCOLOGY

^{67}Ga was first used in 1969 for tumor imaging in patients with Hodgkin disease. ^{67}Ga acts like an iron analogue and circulates in the blood bound to transferrin.

Thallium-201 (^{201}Tl), ^{99m}Tc sestamibi, and ^{99m}Tc tetrofosmin, originally approved for cardiac studies, were found to have tumor-imaging properties. They are taken up by a large number of benign and malignant tumors.

Sentinel lymph-node scintigraphy involves intra-dermal-subcutaneous injection of a radiotracer around the primary lesion, followed by imaging of the lymphatic drainage to the first lymph node. The radiotracer used is ^{99m}Tc-filtered sulphur colloid. An intraoperative gamma probe can provide accurate localization of the node at the time of the surgery.

Indications

Currently ^{67}Ga scan's main clinical use is pretherapy staging and posttherapy evaluation of patients with Hodgkin disease and non-Hodgkin lymphoma. The advances in PET technology and availability are replacing gallium studies in oncology.

[201]Tl is taken up only by viable tumors and can differentiate between posttherapy changes and residual brain tumors. In HIV-positive patients, ^{201}Tl can differentiate between intracerebral malignant lymphomas and infections (e.g., toxoplasmosis). [99m]Tc MIBI is approved for breast imaging.

[111]In-labeled pentetreotide (OctreoScan) is successfully used in imaging amine precursor uptake decarboxylation (APUD)-derived tumors, such as carcinoid, gastrinoma, pheochromocytoma, medullary thyroid cancer, and neuroblastoma.

Lymphoscintigraphy is widely used for the detection of sentinel lymph nodes before surgery for melanoma and breast cancer.

Normal Scintigraphy

Normal scans with the aforementioned agents should demonstrate only the physiologic distribution of the radiotracer. The physiologic ^{67}Ga distribution includes the lacrimal glands, liver, and the bowel (Figure 11-8A).

Abnormal Findings

An abnormal scan is determined by the accumulation of any radiotracer outside its physiologic distribution (Figure 11-8B).

■ CENTRAL NERVOUS SYSTEM

SPECT cerebral perfusion imaging often detects functional abnormalities before structural changes become apparent on anatomic imaging such as CT or MRI. One of the most frequently used radiotracers is ^{99m}Tc HMPAO, which remains retained in the brain for several hours.

Indications

Some of the clinical applications of SPECT cerebral perfusion imaging include detection of acute ischemia, presurgical detection of seizure focus, Alzheimer dementia, and multi-infarct dementia.

[99m]Tc HMPAO and ^{99m}Tc DTPA are used for cerebral flow studies in cases when the patients meet the clinical criteria for brain death, but the electroencephalogram (EEG) is equivocal.

[111]In DTPA is the preferred agent for cysternography. The main clinical applications of this dynamic

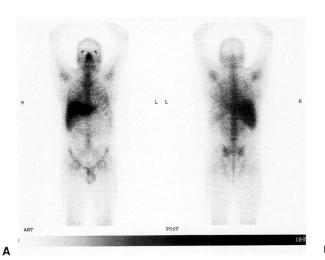

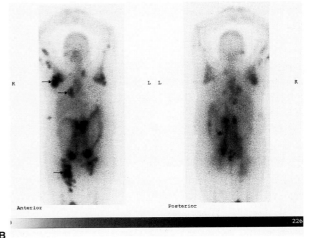

Figure 11-8 • A: Normal ^{67}Ga scan. **B:** [67]Ga scintigraphy showing location of the disease above and below the diaphragm *(arrows)* in a patient with B-cell lymphoma.
(Courtesy of University of Southern California Medical Center, Los Angeles, CA.)

study of the CSF are diagnosis and management of hydrocephalus, assessing the patency of ventriculoperitoneal or ventriculopleural shunts, and determining the site of CSF leaks.

Normal Scintigraphy

Normal studies show uniform distribution of the radiotracer in the brain and the presence of intracerebral blood flow.

Abnormal Findings

Specific radiotracer distribution patterns are described in cerebral ischemia (focal decreased tracer uptake), seizure foci (focal increased tracer accumulation), and dementia (diffuse decreased tracer localization). The absence of intracerebral blood flow is diagnostic for brain death on a cerebral perfusion scintigraphy.

KEY POINTS

1. Characteristic radiotracer distribution patterns are seen in cerebral ischemia, seizure foci, and dementia.
2. Absence of intracerebral blood flow is diagnostic of brain death when the patients meet the clinical criteria, but the electroencephalogram EEG is equivocal.

■ ENDOCRINE

Imaging of the thyroid was one of the first procedures in nuclear medicine after ^{131}I became available to the medical community. Thyroid scintigraphy remains today an essential part of the diagnosis and therapy for thyroid pathology. The radionuclides used are ^{123}I and [131]I. They are concentrated in the thyroid by the sodium-iodine symporter and allow visualization of the gland and calculation of uptake, which is a marker of thyroid function. The normal radioactive iodine uptake in the gland is 5% to 15% at 4 hours and 10% to 30% at 24 hours. For diagnostic studies ^{123}I is preferred because it is a pure gamma emitter and patients are not exposed to beta radiation.

Another application of nuclear medicine in endocrinology is in the identification of parathyroid adenomas and hyperplastic parathyroid glands. It is

important for the surgeon to know the exact location of a parathyroid adenoma before attempting excision. Scintigraphic imaging of the adrenergic nervous system is possible with metaiodobenzylguanidine (MIBG), an analogue of guanethidine, labeled to ^{123}I or [131]I.

Indications

In addition to the diagnosis of various thyroid processes (e.g., Graves disease, thyroiditis, multinodular goiter, cancer), ^{131}I is a safe, efficacious therapy for Graves disease and differentiated thyroid cancer. For a thyroid scintigraphy to be performed, the patient should not have received iodinated contrast agents or solution of potassium iodide (SSKI) or Lugol solution in the 4 to 6 weeks preceding the study because these agents saturate the gland with iodine.

Iodine-labeled MIBG is useful in detecting the location of intra-adrenal paragangliomas, pheochromocytomas, and neuroblastomas. It is important to saturate the thyroid gland with SSKI/Lugol before the study so that radioactive iodine does not get into it. Some drugs (e.g., tricyclic antidepressants, reserpine, guanethidine, labetalol) interfere with MIBG uptake and should be stopped before imaging is performed.

Normal Scintigraphy

Normal thyroid scintigraphy should visualize the butterfly-shaped gland, with homogeneous and uniform radiotracer distribution. No focal radiotracer accumulation outside the thyroid should be seen on a negative parathyroid scan (Figure 11-9A).

Abnormal Findings

Specific patterns of iodine uptake are seen with Graves disease (homogeneous increased uptake, sometimes demonstrating the pyramidal lobe), thyroiditis (usually decreased iodine uptake), multinodular goiter (heterogeneous uptake, areas of hyperfunctioning tissue), and cancer (usually appearing as areas of decreased iodine uptake in comparison with the rest of the gland).

Focal, persistent radiotracer uptake outside the thyroid suggests a parathyroid adenoma on a parathyroid scintigraphy (Figure 11-9B). Its location can be ectopic (i.e., mediastinal).

Imaging the thyroid after ^{131}I cancer ablation therapy allows visualization of the disease and follow-up for recurrence (Figure 11-10).

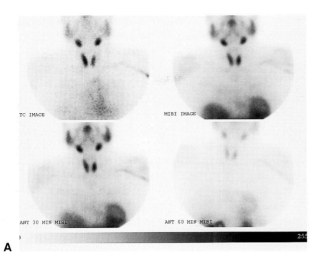

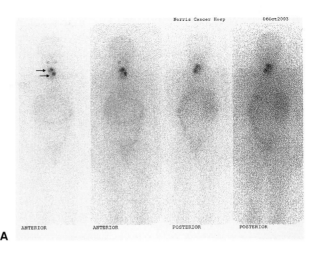

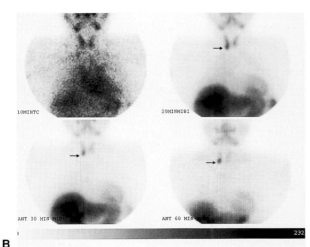

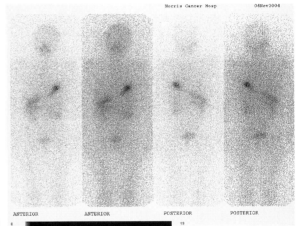

Figure 11-9 • **A:** Normal parathyroid scan. **B:** Parathyroid scan in a patient with right lower parathyroid adenoma *(arrows)*.
(Courtesy of University of Southern California Medical Center, Los Angeles, CA.)

Figure 11-10 • **A:** Whole-body post therapy ^{131}I scan in a patient with metastatic papillary thyroid cancer showing uptake in the thyroid and a cervical lymph node *(arrows)*. **B:** Whole-body follow-up (6 months after therapy) ^{131}I scan in the same patient, indicating resolution of the disease.
(Courtesy of University of Southern California Medical Center, Los Angeles, CA.)

KEY POINTS

1. ^{131}I is an effective diagnostic and therapeutic modality in various thyroid processes.
2. Patient preparation before ^{131}I diagnosis and therapy is essential for a successful procedure.

▓ PET AND MOLECULAR IMAGING

PET is based on coincidence detection of the two gamma rays emitted after a positron and an electron collide and annihilate each other. The product of this annihilation process is two 511-keV gamma rays emitted in opposite directions 180 degrees apart. These rays are detected by paired detectors, and only the coincidence signals are processed by the computer to generate a spatial reconstruction of the original signal.

By far the most widely used positron emitter in clinical practice is F-18 FDG. The other positron emitters available and their physical properties are summarized in Table 11-2.

■ TABLE 11-2

Positron Emitters and Their Physical Characteristics

Radionuclide	Physical Half-Life (min)	Positron Energy (MeV)
Fluorine (F)-18	110	0.635
Rubidium (Rb)-82	1.3	3.15
Carbon (C)-11	20	0.96
Nitrogen (N)-13	10	1.19
Oxygen (O)-15	2	1.73

Current equipment combines a PET with a CT scanner used for attenuation correction and for help in anatomic localization of the lesions.

Molecular imaging is a novel field that provides images that reflect cellular and molecular pathways. It combines the recent tremendous advances of cellular and molecular biology with imaging technologies such as PET, SPECT, digital autoradiography, MRI, magnetic resonance spectroscopy (MRS), optical bioluminescence, optical fluorescence, and ultrasound. New approaches and molecular probes should lead to

better methods for studying biological processes as well as for diagnosing and treating diseases.

Indications

Currently, PET and PET-CT have applications in oncology, cardiology, and brain evaluation. PET scanning has proved to be critical for evaluation of the following types of cancers: lung cancer, breast cancer, thyroid cancer, lymphoma, head and neck cancer, colorectal cancer, and melanoma. Many centers now perform cardiac perfusion and myocardial viability studies using PET. PET is recognized as the major diagnostic imaging modality for Alzheimer dementia.

Normal PET Scan

The normal appearance of a PET scan varies with the radiotracer used. In the case of F-18 FDG (the most commonly used positron emitter), the most intense normal uptake includes the brain, myocardium, kidneys, and urinary bladder (Figure 11-11A). Various physiologic levels of FDG uptake have been described in salivary glands, thyroid, muscles, liver, bowel, uterus, and testicles.

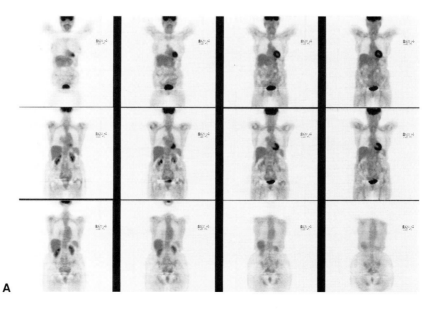

A

Figure 11-11 • A: Normal FDG PET scan showing intense radiotracer accumulation in the brain, myocardium, kidneys, and urinary bladder **B:** PET scan of a patient referred for evaluation of a left lung nodule reveals intense uptake in this lesion *(arrows)*, interpreted as primary lung cancer.
(Courtesy of University of Southern California Medical Center, Los Angeles, CA.)

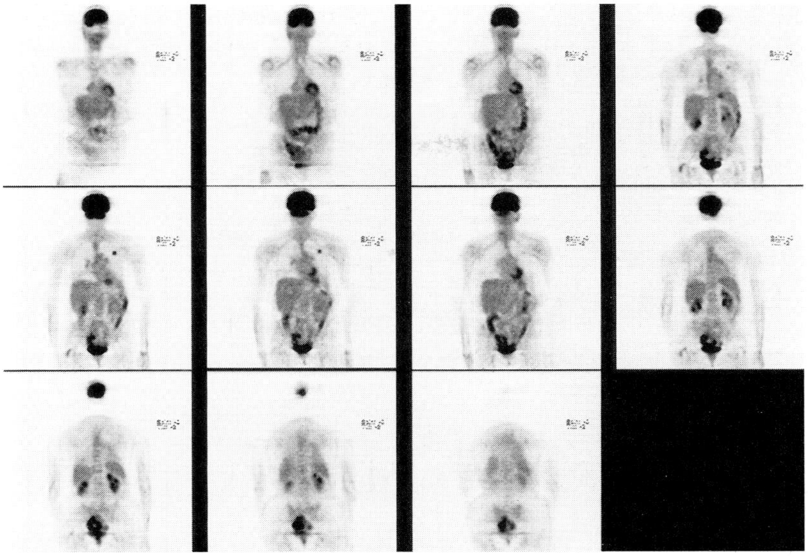

Figure 11-11 · continued

Abnormal PET Scan

F-18 FDG uptake outside its physiologic distribution raises the suspicion of underlying pathology (Figure 11-11B). However, the results should be correlated with anatomic imaging and interpreted in the clinical context.

KEY POINTS
1. PET and molecular imaging offer the ability of better diagnosis and therapy in various pathologic processes.
2. PET-CT is emerging as the most effective tool in the imaging of cancer biology because it combines the anatomic and metabolic-molecular information in a single image.

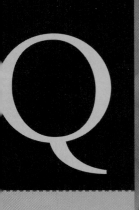

1. A 56-year-old man has a 2-month history of cough, malaise, and weight loss. He has smoked one pack per day for the past 30 years. He denies any fever, chills, or night sweats. What is the next most appropriate diagnostic step?
   A. Chest CT scan
   B. Sputum cultures
   C. PA and lateral chest radiographs
   D. Bronchoscopy
   E. Chest MRI

2. A 20-year-old woman presents to the emergency department following an MVA. She was an unrestrained passenger in a head-on collision and has multiple facial lacerations and contusions. She had been complaining of right hip pain but now is somewhat somnolent with a GCS of 8. What is the next most appropriate diagnostic test?
   A. Contrast-enhanced head CT
   B. Noncontrast head CT
   C. Right-hip radiographs
   D. AP pelvis
   E. Cervical spine radiograph series

3. A 42-year-old man complains of recurrent sinus infections. You treated him 1 month ago with amoxicillin (Clavulanate) for acute sinusitis. He returns stating that although the medication did help, the infection never completely resolved. He affirms that he took the entire course of antibiotics. On physical examination, you notice an effusion behind the right tympanic membrane. What is the most appropriate next step?
   A. Culture the nasopharynx
   B. Prescribe a second course of amoxicillin
   C. Prescribe a course of azithromycin
   D. Order a contrast-enhanced CT of the neck
   E. Order skull radiographs with Waters and Townes views

4. A 74-year-old man presents to the emergency department with slurred speech and left-sided weakness that began 1 hour ago. A noncontrast CT scan of the head reveals an area of hypoattenuation in the right frontal lobe. What is the most likely diagnosis?

   A. Hypertensive crisis
   B. Meningitis
   C. Carotid artery dissection
   D. Stroke
   E. Astrocytoma

5. A 68-year-old man with prostate cancer treated with hormonal suppression presents with low back pain. What is the next step in imaging?
   A. MRI of the spine
   B. X-ray of the spine
   C. Bone scan
   D. CT of the abdomen and pelvis
   E. No imaging study is needed at this time

6. An 8-year-old boy presents to the emergency department with nausea, vomiting, and abdominal pain. An abdominal ultrasound is performed (Figure Q-6): What is the diagnosis?

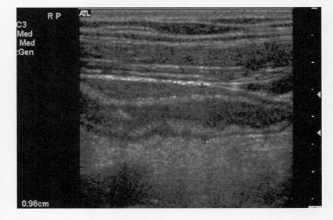

Figure Q-6 • (Courtesy of Cedars-Sinai Medical Center, Los Angeles, CA.)

   A. Crohn disease
   B. Appendicitis
   C. Ulcerative colitis
   D. Small-bowel obstruction
   E. Renal colic

7. A 26-year-old woman presents to the emergency department with left lower quadrant pain and tenderness on examination. Beta-hCG is positive. What is the next most appropriate step in managing this patient?
   A. Inform the patient that she is pregnant, reassure her that the pain is related to the pregnancy, and send her home with arrangements to follow-up with her primary care physician
   B. Obtain a pelvic ultrasound
   C. Perform a speculum examination with a cervical culture
   D. Order an abdominal/pelvic CT scan
   E. Consult obstetrics

8. A 55-year-old woman with a 30 pack-year smoking history is found to have a nodule on a routine CXR. What is the next step in management?
   A. CT of the chest
   B. Chemotherapy
   C. Removal of the nodule
   D. Radiation therapy
   E. PET/CT

9. A 39-year-old woman has intermittent right upper quadrant pain, which is worse after meals. Which of the following ultrasonographic signs is diagnostic of acute cholecystitis?
   A. Fluid around the gallbladder
   B. Thickened gallbladder wall
   C. Gallbladder distension
   D. Gas within the gallbladder wall
   E. Cholelithiasis

10. A 60-year-old man with a history of alcoholism is complaining of intermittent chest pain. A CT scan of the abdomen is shown below (Figure Q-10). What is the most likely diagnosis?

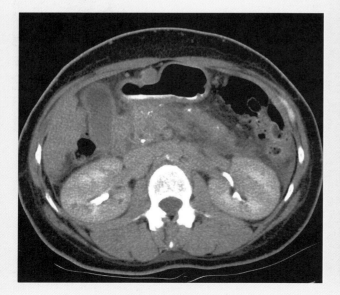

Figure Q-10 • (Courtesy of Cedars-Sinai Medical Center, Los Angeles, CA.)

A. Gastric carcinoma
B. Chronic pancreatitis
C. Renal cell carcinoma
D. Aortic aneurysm
E. Hepatocellular carcinoma

11. A 3-year-old boy presents to the emergency department with cough and difficulty breathing. The mother reports that he has had a fever of 100°F and a barking cough since the night before. A chest radiograph is ordered. Which radiologic sign is most useful in making the diagnosis?
   A. Foreign body in the airway
   B. The steeple sign
   C. Deviated trachea
   D. Unilateral lucent hemithorax
   E. Deep sulcus sign

12. A 55-year-old woman presents to the emergency department for evaluation of right upper quadrant abdominal pain. Abdominal ultrasound shows sludge in the gallbladder. A HIDA scan is ordered, but the gallbladder is not visualized at 1 hour. What statement best describes the situation?
   A. The patient has acute cholecystitis.
   B. The study is not diagnostic, so exploratory laparoscopy is needed.
   C. The patient has cholelithiasis.
   D. IV morphine should be administered to exclude acute cholecystitis.
   E. The study should be repeated the next day.

13. A patient presents with wrist pain status post fall, and a plain film is obtained. In which age group is this injury (Figure Q-13) most likely to occur?

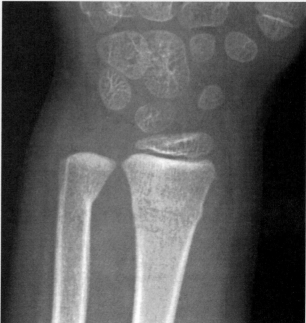

Figure Q-13 • (Courtesy of Cedars-Sinai Medical Center, Los Angeles, CA.)

A. Months
B. 2 years
C. 8 years
D. 20 years
E. 70 years

14. You are called by a nurse in the hospital to evaluate a 65-year-old woman who is 3 days status post hip replacement. She was starting her physical therapy exercises and became short of breath. She is complaining of left-sided chest pain. In this clinical setting, which is the best test to establish the diagnosis?
A. CT scan of the chest with contrast
B. V/Q scan
C. Lower-extremity Doppler examination
D. Angiogram
E. ECG

15. A 35-year-old man presents to the emergency department following a stab wound to the right side of the chest. A CXR reveals blunting of the right costophrenic angle. What is the most likely diagnosis?
A. Pneumothorax
B. Pneumonia
C. Hemopericardium
D. Hemothorax
E. Pulmonary contusion

16. A 35-year-old woman with B-cell lymphoma is admitted to the hospital for chemotherapy. Which of the following is needed before starting Adriamycin?
A. CXR
B. Calculation of EF with MUGA
C. Calculation of EF with echocardiography
D. ECG
E. CT scan of the chest

17. A 46-year-old woman presents with 6 hours of intermittent right flank pain radiating to the groin. Urinalysis shows microscopic hematuria. She has a history of Crohn disease, which has been controlled with steroids in the past. Which of the following is the best test to establish the diagnosis?
A. Barium enema
B. Upper GI series with small-bowel follow-through
C. Noncontrast CT scan of the abdomen and pelvis
D. IVP
E. Ultrasound of the abdomen

18. A 44-year-old woman comes to your office complaining of increasing menstrual bleeding. On physical examination, you determine that the uterus is enlarged and has irregular contours. You suspect that the bleeding is due to uterine leiomyomas. Which is the most appropriate next step in your management?
A. CT scan of the pelvis
B. Ultrasound of the pelvis
C. Abdominal plain radiographs
D. MRI of the pelvis
E. Hysterosalpingogram

19. A 5-year-old child presents with shortness of breath and has previously been diagnosed with asthma. Which of the following radiographic findings should you remember as associated with childhood asthma?
A. Interstitial fibrosis
B. Lobar pneumonia
C. Widened mediastinum
D. Hyperinflated lungs
E. Pneumothorax

20. A 1-day-old girl presents from the nursery with frequent vomiting and abdominal bloating. An abdominal radiograph is obtained (Figure Q-20). What is the diagnosis?

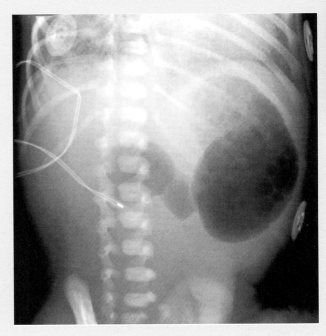

Figure Q-20 • (Courtesy of Cedars-Sinai Medical Center, Los Angeles, CA.)

A. Pyloric stenosis
B. Duodenal atresia
C. Necrotizing enterocolitis
D. Hirschsprung disease
E. Tracheoesophageal fistula

21. A 69-year-old woman has a history of peripheral vascular disease. Which of the following lesions is most amenable to percutaneous intervention?

A. A 3-cm stenosis of the popliteal artery immediately above the knee joint

B. A 4-cm occlusion of the popliteal artery extending across the knee joint

C. An 8-cm stenosis of the peroneal and anterior tibial arteries with reconstitution of flow in the distal vessels near the ankle joint

D. Several 2- to 4-cm stenoses of the popliteal, anterior tibial and posterior tibial arteries

E. A 7-cm stenosis of the superficial femoral artery

22. A 42-year-old man with recent MI is evaluated before CABG. What is the best method to assess the presence of viable myocardium before revascularization?
    A. F-18 FDG cardiac PET
    B. ECG
    C. Cardiac SPECT
    D. Cardiac catheterization
    E. Transthoracic echocardiography

23. A 33-year-old man presents with abdominal pain, nausea, and vomiting. His blood alcohol level is elevated. A KUB is obtained and shows an ileus and sentinel loop in the left upper quadrant. What is the most likely diagnosis?
    A. Diverticulitis
    B. High-grade small-bowel obstruction
    C. Sigmoid volvulus
    D. Acute pancreatitis
    E. Crohn disease

24. A 64-year-old woman presents to your office with complaints of joint pain and stiffness in the hands and wrists. You notice mild arthritis and ulnar deviation of bilateral MCP joints and order plain radiographs of the hands and wrists. The films reveal multiple bilateral periarticular joint erosions. What is the most likely diagnosis?
    A. Gout
    B. Pseudogout
    C. Chronic osteomyelitis
    D. Rheumatoid arthritis
    E. Osteoarthritis

25. A 75-year-old woman who is on chronic warfarin therapy for atrial fibrillation presents to the emergency department after falling from a stepladder. She complains of dizziness and headache. She denies loss of consciousness. A head CT is obtained (Figure Q-25). What is the diagnosis?
    A. Epidural hematoma
    B. Subdural hematoma
    C. Subarachnoid hemorrhage
    D. Lymphoma
    E. Metastatic lesion

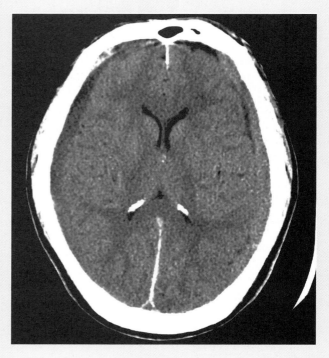

Figure Q-25 • (Courtesy of Cedars-Sinai Medical Center, Los Angeles, CA.)

26. A 2-year-old child is brought to the emergency department by her mother because the child became tachypneic suddenly while eating. On examination, the child is restless, grunting, and using accessory muscles to breathe. Respiratory rate is 40 per minute. Temperature is 37.1°C. What findings are expected on the CXR?
    A. Hyperinflated right lung
    B. Alveolar opacification in a lobar distribution
    C. Large, spiculated mass
    D. Blunting of the costophrenic angle on one side
    E. No abnormal findings

27. A 33-year-old man presents to the emergency department with right-sided back pain that radiates to the right groin. The pain began 2 hours ago and is relatively constant in intensity. Microscopic hematuria is found on laboratory examination. What is the most appropriate imaging test at this time?
    A. Ultrasound
    B. IVP
    C. CT urogram
    D. KUB
    E. MRI of the abdomen

28. A 60-year-old man presents to your office with a chief complaint of left facial swelling and progressive left-sided facial droop for the past 3 months. You order an imaging study, which is shown in Figure Q-28. What is the most likely diagnosis?
    A. Mumps
    B. Parotid carcinoma

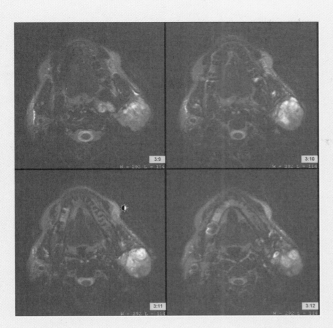

Figure Q-28 • (Courtesy of Cedars-Sinai Medical Center, Los Angeles, CA.)

C. Stroke
D. Parapharyngeal abscess
E. Pleomorphic adenoma

29. A 59-year-old man presents to your office complaining of left-sided weakness and recurrent headaches for the past month. You order a CT scan of the head, shown below (Figure Q-29). What is the most likely diagnosis?

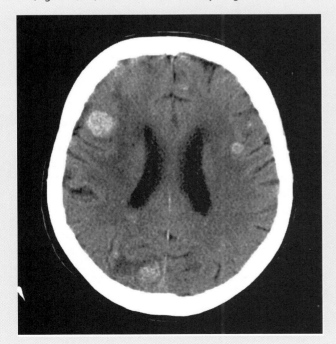

Figure Q-29 • (Courtesy of Cedars-Sinai Medical Center, Los Angeles, CA.)

A. Abscesses
B. Intracerebral hematomas
C. Multiple sclerosis
D. Metastases
E. Glioblastoma multiforme

30. A 63-year-old woman with a history of ovarian cancer presents to the emergency department with abdominal pain and nausea. Supine and upright abdominal films are shown below (Figure Q-30A, B). What is the most likely diagnosis?

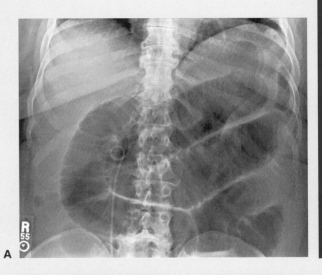

A

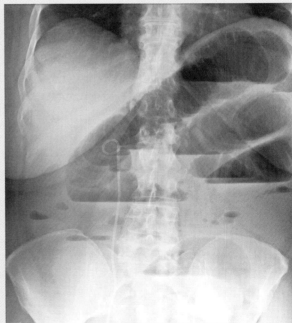

B

Figure Q-30 A, B • (Courtesy of Cedars-Sinai Medical Center, Los Angeles, CA.)

A. Paralytic ileus
B. Small-bowel obstruction
C. Colonic obstruction
D. Pancreatitis with sentinel loop
E. Fecal impaction

31. A 45-year-old woman is brought in by ambulance after an automobile accident. The initial CXR is obtained (Figure Q-31). What is the next appropriate step in patient management?

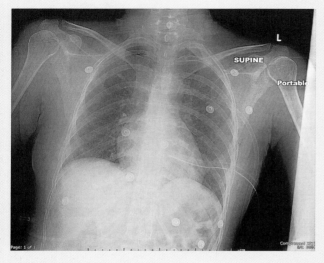

Figure Q-31 • (Courtesy of University of Southern California Medical Center, Los Angeles, CA.)

A. Take the patient to the operating room for exploration
B. Follow up with another CXR to determine whether a pneumothorax is developing
C. Order an emergent chest CT scan with IV contrast
D. Order a rib series to evaluate for fractures
E. Place bilateral chest tubes

32. A 2-year-old boy presents with intermittent, crampy abdominal pain. You order an upright film of the abdomen to evaluate for possible pneumoperitoneum (Figure Q-32). What is the diagnosis?
A. Acute gastroenteritis
B. Intussusception
C. Appendicitis
D. Bowel obstruction
E. Pneumoperitoneum

33. You are asked for advice regarding the best modality to evaluate a pregnant patient suspected to have a PE. What is the best advice?
A. To perform CTPA because it involves the lowest radiation
B. To order a V/Q scan with half the usual dose of radiotracer
C. To start anticoagulation therapy
D. Recommend bed rest
E. Request placement of an IVC filter

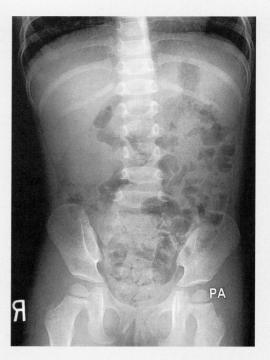

Figure Q-32 • (Courtesy of University of Southern California Medical Center, Los Angeles, CA.)

34. A 22-year-old woman presents with increasing left knee pain. The anterior view of the knee is shown in Figure Q-34. What is the most likely diagnosis?

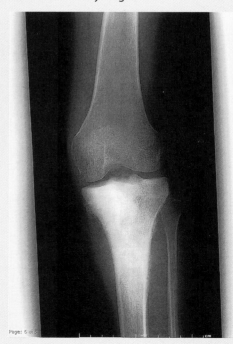

Figure Q-34 • (Courtesy of University of Southern California Medical Center, Los Angeles, CA.)

A. Septic arthritis
B. Rheumatoid arthritis
C. Osteomyelitis
D. Osteosarcoma
E. Old fracture

35. A 75-year-old man presents with difficulty urinating. An image from the contrast-enhanced CT of the abdomen and pelvis is shown in Figure Q-35. What is the most likely cause of the circumferential urinary bladder wall thickening?

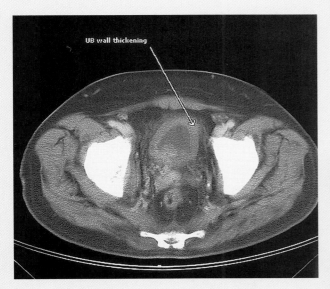

Figure Q-35 • (Courtesy of University of Southern California Medical Center, Los Angeles, CA.)

A. Urinary bladder transitional cell carcinoma
B. Outlet obstruction by an enlarged prostate
C. Metastatic disease
D. Conus medullaris syndrome
E. Prostate carcinoma

36. A 67-year-old man presents with an elevated PSA and an indurated prostate on physical examination. The CT obtained as part of the workup is shown in Figure Q-36. What is the next appropriate imaging step?
A. Bone scintigraphy to evaluate for bone metastases
B. Whole-body MRI
C. Repeat CT scan for follow-up
D. Plain films of the spine
E. CXR

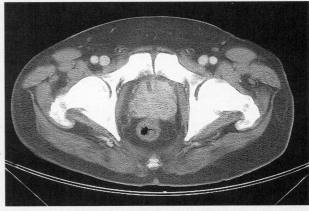

Figure Q-36 • (Courtesy of University of Southern California Medical Center, Los Angeles, CA.)

37. A 43-year-old woman presents to the emergency department complaining of chest pain radiating to her back, worsened with deep inspiration. You decide to perform a CT (Figure Q-37). What is the diagnosis?

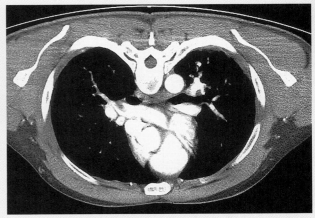

Figure Q-37 • (Courtesy of University of Southern California Medical Center, Los Angeles, CA.)

A. Aortic dissection
B. Spontaneous pneumothorax
C. Septic pulmonary emboli
D. Rib fractures
E. Bland PE

38. A 56-year-old man is admitted for evaluation of chest pain. What is the indication to perform a stress cardiac scintigraphy?
A. Family history of dyslipidemia
B. Risk stratification after MI

C. Normal exercise stress test
D. Ruling out MI
E. Age and sex

39. A 22-year-old man presents with acute onset of short-ness of breath, without any history of trauma. The CXR demonstrates a right-sided pneumothorax and no other abnormalities. If the pneumothorax is to recur or not improve on treatment, what would be the next imaging step?
   A. Order a bone scan in search for a primary osteosarcoma
   B. Obtain a rib series to identify any traumatic fractures, even though the patient denies any injury
   C. Order a CT of the chest
   D. Perform an MRI of the chest
   E. Ask for an echocardiogram

40. An 18-year-old man comes to the office complaining of frontal headaches, fever, and nasal congestion. He has undergone a course of antibiotic therapy, but symptoms have worsened. You decide to obtain imaging to evalu-ate the extent of disease. Which modality will you choose?
   A. A plain film series of the sinuses
   B. An MRI of the brain
   C. A noncontrast CT of the sinuses
   D. A skull nuclear medicine scintigraphy
   E. An ultrasound of the sinuses

41. A 46-year-old woman with known breast carcinoma presents with focal neurologic deficits. Which is the best imaging modality to evaluate for possible brain metastases?
   A. CT of the brain with IV contrast
   B. MRI of the brain with contrast
   C. Nuclear medicine whole-body scintigraphy
   D. Plain radiographs of the skull
   E. CT of the brain without IV contrast

42. A 23-year-old woman presents with acute left lower quad-rant pain and beta-hCG level of 3500 mIU/mL. A trans-vaginal ultrasound is obtained, but no ectopic or intrauterine pregnancy could be identified. What is your conclusion?
   A. An ectopic pregnancy is excluded.
   B. The conceptus is too small to be visualized.
   C. CT of the pelvis should be obtained.
   D. The diagnosis is a completed spontaneous abortion.
   E. An ectopic pregnany cannot be excluded.

43. A 44-year-old woman presents with acute right upper quadrant pain, worse after meals. Acute cholecystitis is sus-pected clinically. A right upper quadrant ultrasound is ordered for confirmation (Figure Q-43). What does the image show?

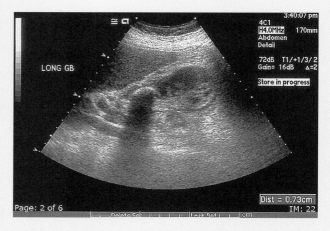

Figure Q-43 • (Courtesy of University of Southern California Medical Center, Los Angeles, CA.)

   A. Gas within the gallbladder wall
   B. Gas within the gallbladder lumen
   C. Cholelithiasis and gallbladder wall thickening
   D. Cholelithiasis, but normal gallbladder wall thickness
   E. Normal gallbadder

44. A 67-year-old man with known cirrhosis presents with decompensated ascites. You suspect portal vein throm-bosis as the etiology. Which is the best first-line test to order?
   A. CT with IV contrast
   B. MRI with sequences to detect color flow
   C. Portal vein conventional angiogram
   D. Doppler ultrasound of the portal vein
   E. Grayscale ultrasound

45. An 18-month-old child is brought to the hospital with col-icky, intermittent abdominal pain and currant jelly stools. What radiologic test would you first order?
   A. CT of the abdomen with IV contrast
   B. An ultrasound of the abdomen
   C. An MRI of the abdomen
   D. A plain radiograph of the abdomen, upright or cross-table lateral
   E. CXR

46. A 26-year-old woman is found to have a thyroid nodule at a routine health examination in her doctor's office. What is the most significant risk factor for this nodule to be thy-roid cancer?

A. Age
B. Sex
C. External radiation to the neck area as a child
D. Diet
E. No risk factors are associated with adult thyroid cancer.

47. A thyroid scintigraphy shows a cold nodule correspon-
ding to one palpated on physical examination. Biopsy shows
papillary thyroid carcinoma. What is the best threapeutic
approach?
A. Chemotherapy
B. External beam radiation
C. Surgical excision
D. Surgical excision followed by I-131 ablation
E. Hormonal suppression of the thyroid

48. A 21-year-old man was brought to the emergency
department with a gunshot wound to the chest. CT did
not demonstrate any vascular injury, and the patient
is awake and stable. You are concerned that an
esophageal injury occurred. Which test would you
order?
A. An esophagogram with Gastrografin (oral contrast)
B. An esophagogram with barium
C. An esophagogram with water
D. Do not order any radiographic tests at this time and
observe patient
E. Consider returning patient for esophagogram as out-
patient

49. A 58-year-old man with diabetes mellitus describes a
1-month history of a nonhealing ulcer of the right foot
draining pus. A right foot x-ray series demonstrates no
abnormality other than the soft-tissue defect. What is the
next step?
A. Send the patient home on a trial of oral antibiotics
B. Obtain follow up x-ray of the foot in 1 week
C. Plan a short course of IV antibiotics
D. Order an MRI or bone scan of the foot to evaluate for
osteomyelitis
E. Plan amputation of the involved area

50. A 38-year-old woman who underwent liver transplant sur-
gery 2 days ago develops signs of hypovolemia. You are
not certain of the bleeding site (it might be at the anasto-
mosis) and order what?
A. CT scan of the abdomen with IV contrast
B. CT scan of the abdomen with oral contrast
C. Abdominal X-ray
D. GI bleeding scan
E. Angiography

51. A 47-year-old woman is brought in by ambulance after
an MVA. A pneumothorax was identified on the initial
CXR and a chest tube was placed in the right pleural cavity. The patient is stable, so you obtain a delayed upright
follow-up CXR (Figure Q-51). What does the plain film
show?

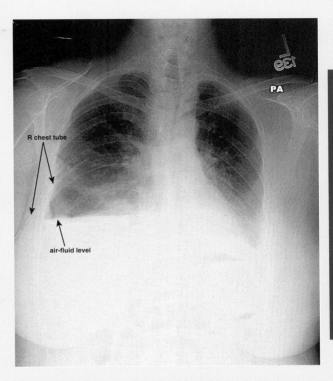

Figure Q-51 • (Courtesy of University of Southern California Medical
Center, Los Angeles, CA.)

A. A widened mediastinum suspicious for vascular injury
B. A right pleural space chest tube, and no other abnor-
mality
C. Lung collapse
D. Right lower lobe pneumonia
E. A right pleural space chest tube and a right hydro-
pneumothorax

52. A 3-year-old boy presents with urinary tract infection.
After an ultrasound demonstrated normal urinary tract
anatomy, a VCUG is ordered (Figure Q-52). What does it
show?
A. Normal outline of the urinary tract
B. A distended urinary bladder but mild reflux
C. Severe vesicoureteral reflux
D. Ureteral obstruction
E. Urethral obstruction

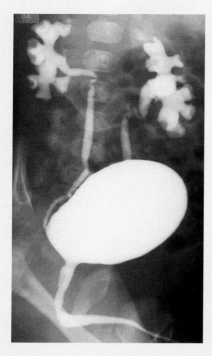

Figure Q-52 • (Reprinted with permission from Patel, P.R. Lecture Notes: Radiology. Oxford: Blackwell Publishing, 2005.)

53. A 22-year-old woman presents with left lower quadrant pain and a positive pregnancy test. On the pelvic ultrasound obtained (Figure Q-53), the white arrow points to a normal uterus, and the cursors outline what?

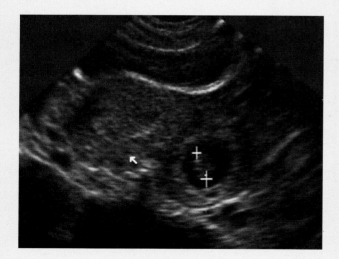

Figure Q-53 • (Reprinted with permission from Patel, P.R. Lecture Notes: Radiology. Oxford: Blackwell Publishing, 2005.)

A. Intrauterine pregnancy
B. Ovarian neoplasm
C. Dilated fallopian tube

D. An inflamed appendix
E. An ectopic pregnancy

54. A 59-year-old man complains of fever and worsening cough for 2 weeks. You obtain a CXR (Figure Q-54). What does the film show, and what will you do next?

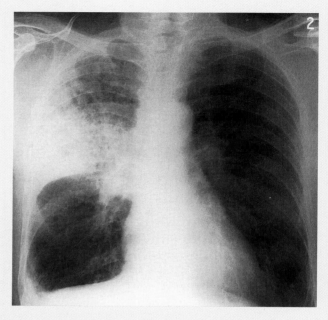

Figure Q-54 • (Reprinted with permission from Patel, P.R. Lecture Notes: Radiology. Oxford: Blackwell Publishing, 2005.)

A. The film shows an artifact over the right chest, and redo of the film is needed.
B. CXR shows a right upper lobe infiltrate, so treatment and a 6-week follow-up film for resolution are warranted.
C. The film shows right upper lobe collapse and bronchoscopy should be done.
D. No definite abnormality is appreciated, and no action should be taken.
E. The film shows pulmonary contusion and follow-up is needed.

55. A 27-year-old woman complains of pelvic discomfort. Her last menstrual period was 2 weeks ago. Her physical examination is normal, and a pelvic ultrasound is remarkable only for the following findings (Figure Q-55). You explain to the patient that these findings are what?

A. Compatible with a normal midcycle ovary
B. Suggestive of ovarian cancer
C. Exemplary of a mass with thickened walls and internal septations

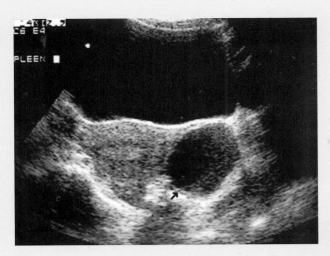

Figure Q-55 • (Reprinted with permission from Patel, P.R. Lecture Notes: Radiology. Oxford: Blackwell Publishing, 2005.)

D. Further imaging with a pelvic MRI is required
E. Consistent with ovarian metastases

56. A 45-year-old man with history of alcohol abuse presents with severe abdominal pain to the emergency department. After analgesics he is able to stand briefly for an upright CXR (Figure Q-56). What does the film show?

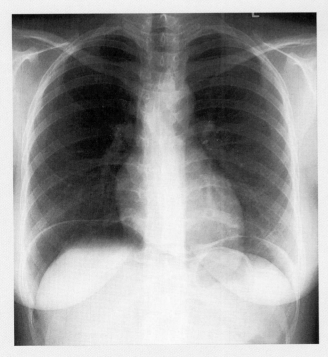

Figure Q-56 • (Reprinted with permission from Patel, P.R. Lecture Notes: Radiology. Oxford: Blackwell Publishing, 2005.)

A. No abnormality
B. Lower-lobe pneumonia
C. An enlarged heart
D. Moderate-volume pneumoperitoneum
E. Rib fractures

57. A 33-year-old woman complains of heavy menstrual periods. Urine pregnancy test is negative and physical examination reveals a slightly enlarged uterus. Pelvic ultrasound is shown below (Figure Q-57). What is the most likely diagnosis?

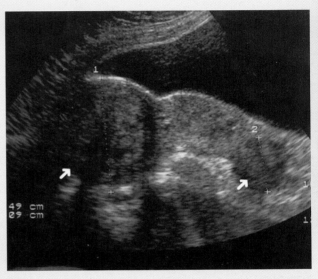

Figure Q-57 • (Reprinted with permission from Patel, P.R. Lecture Notes: Radiology. Oxford: Blackwell Publishing, 2005.)

A. Tubo-ovarian abscess
B. Uterine fibroids
C. Ectopic pregnancy
D. Cervicitis
E. Ovarian cyst

58. A 67-year-old man presents with left lower quadrant abdominal pain. You obtain contrast-enhanced CT of the abdomen and pelvis and notice the renal lesions (Figure Q-58). What would you do next?
A. Obtain a urology surgical consult for removal of lesions
B. Order a renal ultrasound to ensure the lesions have similar appearance
C. Reassure the patient that the lesions represent benign renal cysts
D. Obtain a nephrology consult to assess the renal function
E. Order a follow-up CT scan

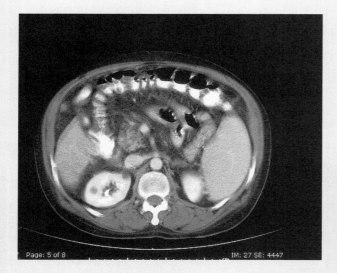

Figure Q-58 • (Courtesy of University of Southern California Medical Center, Los Angeles, CA.)

59. A 49-year-old woman presents with 3 days of severe epigastric pain. You obtain a CT of the abdomen (Figure Q-59) without contrast because the creatinine level is elevated (2.3). Based on the findings, what other imaging should you obtain?

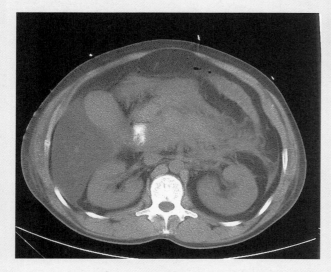

Figure Q-59 • (Courtesy of University of Southern California Medical Center, Los Angeles, CA.)

A. CT shows acute pancreatitis, and no other imaging is indicated

B. An ultrasound to evaluate for choledocholithiasis as the cause of pancreatitis

C. MRCP to evaluate for choledocholithiasis

D. HIDA scan

E. Plain film of the abdomen (KUB) to confirm stones

60. A 5-year-old boy is brought in due to worsening headaches and vomiting. The sagittal image from the MRI you ordered (Figure Q-60) shows what?

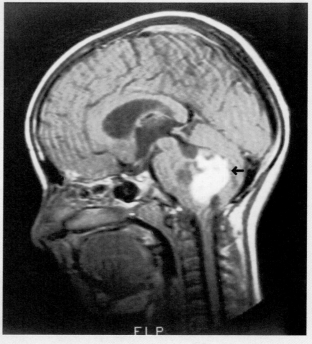

Figure Q-60 • (Reprinted with permission from Patel, P.R. Lecture Notes: Radiology. Oxford: Blackwell Publishing, 2005).

A. Normal anatomy and arrow points to the fourth ventricle

B. Enlarged, obstructed fourth ventricle

C. A cyst in the fourth ventricle

D. An old infarct

E. Arrow points to a mass in the fourth ventricle

61. A 77-year-old woman presents to the emergency department with shortness of breath. The CXR (Figure Q-61) reveals what?

A. Normal chest

B. Pneumothorax

C. Rib fractures

D. Congestive heart failure

E. Large pleural effusions

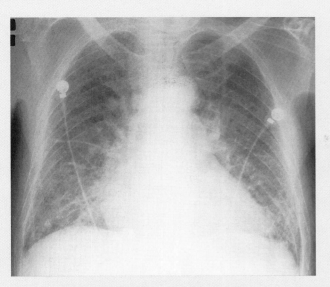

Figure Q-61 • (Reprinted with permission from Patel, P.R. Lecture Notes: Radiology. Oxford: Blackwell Publishing, 2005.)

62. A 67-year-old man is complaining of headaches that have worsened in the last month. You obtain a CT of the brain without intravenous contrast to exclude intracranial hemorrhage. What does the image (Figure Q-62) show?

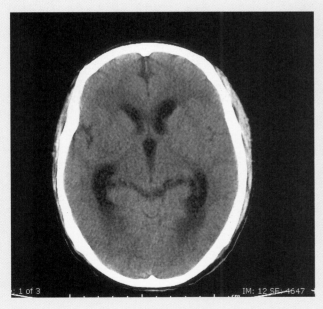

Figure Q-62 • (Courtesy of University of Southern California Medical Center, Los Angeles, CA.)

   A. Dilated ventricles
   B. Intraventricular hemorrhage
   C. No abnormality

D. Subdural hematoma
E. Intraparenchymal hemorrhage

63. When hydrocephalus is diagnosed on a CT scan, what should be your concern, and what other imaging test would you order?
   A. Patient may have suffered trauma and a repeat CT scan should be obtained to evaluate for delayed hemorrhage.
   B. A central nervous system (CNS) tumor needs to be excluded, and an MRI of the brain needs to be ordered.
   C. The CT scan was normal, and no further imaging is necessary.
   D. The patient may have suffered an ischemic stroke that does not yet show on this CT scan, so a delayed scan or an MRI with diffusion-weighted sequence needs to be obtained.
   E. The patient may have an occult fracture, and a skull x-ray is indicated.

64. The barium study obtained on a 35-year-old man with persistent lower abdominal pain, diarrhea, and fever is seen on Figure Q-64. The arrows point to the findings. What is the most likely diagnosis?

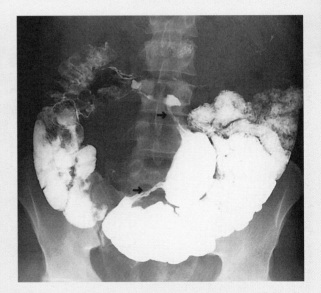

Figure Q-64 • (Reprinted with permission from Patel, P.R. Lecture Notes: Radiology. Oxford: Blackwell Publishing, 2005).

   A. Parasitic infestation
   B. A mass displacing bowel
   C. Small-bowel obstruction
   D. Crohn disease
   E. No abnormality is really present

65. A 49-year-old man was intubated after head trauma. You are shown the CXR obtained post endotracheal tube (ETT) placement (Figure Q-65). What are the CXR findings?

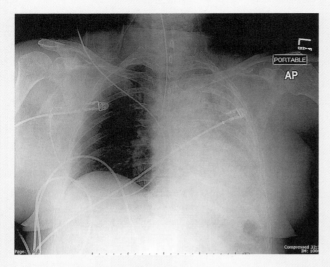

Figure Q-65 • (Courtesy of University of Southern California Medical Center, Los Angeles, CA.)

A. The ETT is in the esophagus.
B. The ETT is in good position.
C. The patient has left-sided pneumonia.
D. A large left pleural effusion is present.
E. The ETT is too low so the left lung is collapsed.

66. A 25-year-old woman who is 16 weeks pregnant presents with sudden onset of shortness of breath and pleuritic chest pain. Trying to limit the radiation exposure, you obtain the V/Q scan in Figure Q-66. What does the image show?

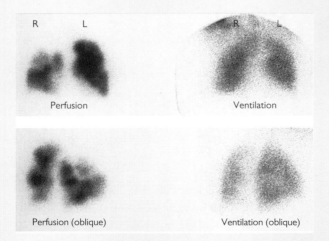

Figure Q-66 • (Reprinted with permission from Patel, P.R. Lecture Notes: Radiology. Oxford: Blackwell Publishing, 2005).

A. V/Q scan demonstrates V/Q mismatch caused by PE.
B. V/Q scan demonstrates V/Q mismatch caused by air trapping in this patient, who has asthma.
C. V/Q scan is normal (no V/Q mismatch).
D. The test results are indeterminate.
E. The heterogeneity of perfusion is due to artifact.

67. When a V/Q mismatch is identified, what would you do next?
A. Treat the patient for pulmonary emboli
B. Treat the patient for acute asthma
C. Reassure the patient she does not have emboli and discharge her home
D. Obtain a pulmonary angiogram
E. Remove the metal pad overlying the patient that created the artifact

68. A 72-year-old man presents with mild upper abdominal pain. You palpated a pulsatile abdominal mass and ordered a CT of chest and abdomen with IV contrast (Figure Q-68). What is the diagnosis?

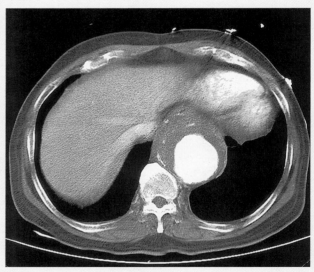

Figure Q-68 • (Courtesy of University of Southern California Medical Center, Los Angeles, CA.)

A. Epigastric mass
B. Hiatal hernia
C. Thoracoabdominal aortic aneurysm
D. No abnormality present
E. Ventricular aneurysm due to MI

69. When an enlarged IV contrast-filled structure is identified in the retroperitoneum, what is the next step in management?
A. Refer the patient to the surgery service for removal of tumor
B. A Nissen fundoplication should be performed to correct the hiatal hernia

C. Refer the patient for surgical evaluation for aortic aneurysm repair

D. Reassure the patient and discharge him home

E. Evaluate the patient for second episode of MI

70. A 77-year-old man complains of severe back pain. Multiple lytic lesions were seen in the pelvis and spine on the lumbar spine series. While waiting for serum protein electrophoresis, you decide to get more imaging for faster preliminary diagnosis. Which test would you order?

A. Bone scintigraphy (bone scan)

B. MRI of the spine

C. CT scan of the spine

D. Metastatic skeletal survey

E. Repeat the spine x-ray

71. A 42-year-old man with a history of an MVA and intracranial hemorrhage develops right lower extremity swelling and edema. Doppler ultrasound reveals DVT extending from the midsuperficial femoral vein to the infrarenal IVC. What should be the appropriate position of an IVC filter in this patient?

A. Immediately superior to the most proximal aspect of the thrombus

B. In the infrarenal IVC with the proximal tip of the filter just below the level of the renal veins

C. With the midportion of the filter at the level of the renal veins

D. Immediately superior to the level of the renal veins

E. Immediately inferior to the right atrium

72. A 54-year-old woman with squamous cell cancer of the cervix is found to have hydronephrosis of the left kidney on ultrasound examination. During placement of a percutaneous nephrostomy tube, what is the ideal location for the entrance point of the tube?

A. Anterior calyx

B. Renal pelvis

C. Posterior calyx

D. Lateral aspect of the renal parenchyma

E. Proximal ureter

73. A 61-year-old man with biliary obstruction secondary to cholangiocarinoma is to have a percutaneous biliary drainage catheter placed by interventional radiology. Before the procedure, which of the following is the most important laboratory value to confirm?

A. Hemoglobin

B. INR

C. Total bilirubin

D. Direct bilirubin

E. ESR

74. A 22-year-old man presents to the emergency department after a motorcycle accident. CXR reveals widening of the mediastinum. What is the most probable location of the posttraumatic pseudoaneurysm?

A. Origin of the brachiocephalic artery

B. Root of the aorta

C. At the level of the diaphragm

D. At the level of the ligamentum arteriosum

E. There are several sites throughout the thoracic aorta at which traumatic pseudoaneurysms occur with relatively equal frequency.

75. A 57-year-old man complains of claudication of the buttock and impotence. On physical examination, he is found to have diminished femoral pulses. What is the most likely etiology of his disease?

A. Mycotic aneurysm

B. Takayasu arteritis

C. Posttraumatic pseudoaneurysm

D. Marfan syndrome

E. Atherosclerotic disease

A Answers

1. C (Chapter 4)

The PA and lateral chest radiographs are the most useful screening tests in suspected thoracic disease. In this case, the diagnosis is most likely lung cancer, which most likely will be detected by the PA and lateral radiographs. Although the chest CT may be useful in staging, it is not an effective screening tool. Sputum cultures would be more useful if the patient had fevers or chills. Bronchoscopy is invasive and is not indicated as a screening tool. Chest MRI is not useful in suspected lung parenchymal disease. It is very useful in looking at the heart and mediastinum. Confirmation of suspected lung cancer diagnosis is obtained by either transthoracic biopsy under CT guidance or by bronchoscopy.

2. B (Chapter 3)

The most appropriate diagnostic test in head trauma with altered level of consciousness is a noncontrast CT scan of the head. Epidural and subdural hematomas are life-threatening and can easily be excluded by noncontrast head CT. A contrast-enhanced head CT is not indicated in trauma because the contrast can mask hemorrhage. Diagnosis of pelvic injury is secondary to intracranial injury. Cervical spine series is indicated, especially if the patient has neck pain; however, the patient can be stabilized in a neck collar until after the head CT.

3. D (Chapter 2)

In adults with recurrent sinus infections or otitis media, there is an increased incidence of a mass causing an obstruction to the normal drainage from the sinuses and nasal passages. A CT scan of the neck will show the anatomy and rule out any head and neck mass. Skull radiographs are an acceptable screening test for sinusitis but are not useful for excluding head and neck masses.

4. D (Chapter 3)

Hypoattenuation in a vascular distribution is the hallmark of stroke. Combined with the clinical presentation, the patient likely had a right MCA stroke. Hypertension may cause similar symptoms, but radiographically it presents as an intra-parenchymal hemorrhage, most often in the basal ganglia. Meningitis is not detectable by noncontrast CT, although this could show secondary signs such as hydrocephalus. Carotid artery dissection could present in this way, but less commonly. Astrocytoma would appear as a soft-tissue mass surrounded by a ring of low-attenuation edema.

5. C (Chapter 11)

The patient probably has bone metastasis to the spine. Evaluation with a whole-body bone scan to determine the extent of disease is the best option. An MRI of the spine, a spine x-ray, or x-ray of the abdomen and pelvis can detect some bone lesions, but these modalities do not have the same sensitivity as a bone scan. A patient with prostate cancer presenting with low back pain needs imaging studies to exclude bone metastasis as the cause of the symptoms.

6. B (Chapter 5)

The ultrasound reveals a dilated appendix containing a calcified appendicolith at its proximal end. In children, ultrasound is the preferred test for the diagnosis of appendicitis because of the lack of ionizing radiation.

7. B (Chapter 7)

Although the beta-hCG is positive, a normal intrauterine pregnancy is not guaranteed. An ectopic pregnancy may be the cause of the abdominal pain. A CT scan is contraindicated because of the potentially harmful effects of ionizing radiation to the fetus.

8. E (Chapter 11)

PET/CT is the most useful imaging tool for assessing the presence of additional lesions in solitary lung nodules found on CXR or CT. Starting therapy (chemotherapy, surgery, or radiation therapy) before knowing the extent of disease is not common medical practice.

9. D (Chapter 5)

The presence of gas within the gallbladder wall represents acute gangrenous cholecystitis. Pericholecystic fluid, gallbladder-wall thickening, stones, and gallbladder distension are all findings associated with (although not diagnostic of) acute cholecystitis. For these radiologic findings, clinical correlation should be used to confirm the diagnosis. Other conditions may cause gallbladder wall thickening (i.e., hepatitis A, hypoalbuminemia).

10. B (Chapter 5)

The CT section through the upper abdomen reveals calcifications within the pancreas and inflammation of the peripancreatic mesenteric fat. Pancreatitis classically presents as upper abdominal pain that radiates through to the back; however, some patients may describe it as chest pain.

11. B (Chapter 9)

The clinical presentation is of croup, which is associated with the steeple sign, or a tapering of the trachea on the frontal chest radiograph.

12. D (Chapter 11)

It is not unusual to have no scintigraphic evidence of gallbladder at 1 hour in a HIDA scan. To rule out acute cholecystitis, morphine should be administered because it contracts the sphincter of Oddi and the radiotracer excreted by the liver should fill the gallbladder. No visualization of the gallbladder after morphine administration or at 4 hours after the study was started is consistent with the diagnosis of acute cholecystitis. Acute cholecystitis and cholelithiasis are certainly on the differential diagnosis list, but they are not proven yet. There is no reason to repeat the study the following morning.

13. C (Chapter 8)

The radiograph of the wrist reveals a torus fracture of the radial metaphysis. This is associated with a fall onto an outstretched hand in a child 5 to 10 years old. A 2-month-old would have a bowing type deformity after trauma. A 2-year-old would most likely have a greenstick-type fracture. An adult would likely have a Colles fracture.

14. B (Chapter 4)

A V/Q scan is the least invasive test that will give the most diagnostic information. Although the gold standard for diagnosing pulmonary embolus, a conventional pulmonary angiogram is an invasive procedure and therefore not a first choice. A routine CT of the chest with IV contrast does **not** time the imaging for the contrast to be maximally concentrated within the pulmonary arteries (whereas a CT pulmonary angiogram does).

15. D (Chapter 4)

Blunting of the costophrenic angle is a sign of pleural fluid. Following a penetrating wound to the chest, the fluid is most likely blood.

16. B (Chapter 11)

Adriamycin is potentially cardiotoxic, and assessment of ejection fraction (EF) prior to chemotherapy is needed. MUGA is the most precise imaging tool used for calculation of EF. A CT of the chest has no place for evaluating the ejection fraction. More recently cardiac MRI has gained some ground for this purpose.

17. C (Chapter 6)

The diagnosis is nephrolithiasis. The patient's history of Crohn disease is a predisposing factor for developing renal calculi and the microscopic hematuria distinguishes the pain from a gastrointestinal etiology. An IVP could also establish the diagnosis, but in the emergency department situation the noncontrast CT scan is the more appropriate test because of the decreased radiation exposure and lack of risk from administration of intravenous iodine contrast.

18. B (Chapter 7)

An ultrasound will reveal uterine leiomyomas as hypoechoic areas, which may be mucosal, subserosal, or serosal. An MRI will also provide diagnostic information but is generally not used as a screening test; rather, it is used if diagnostic questions remain after ultrasound.

19. D (Chapter 4)

Hyperinflation of the lungs and peribronchial inflammation are nonspecific radiologic findings associated with childhood asthma.

20. B (Chapter 9)

The radiograph reveals a "double-bubble" sign, with two large air bubbles in the upper abdomen. These air bubbles represent air in the stomach and duodenal bulb.

21. A (Chapter 10)

Focal lesions that are less than 5 cm long are ideal for percutaneous intervention. Multifocal or longer lesions are better suited for surgical treatment. If a stent is to be placed percutaneously, it is undesirable to position one across a joint.

22. A (Chapter 11)

There is evidence that assessment of myocardial metabolism with F-18 FDG PET is the best modality for identification of viable myocardium prior to revascularization with CABG. Cardiac SPECT with ^{201}Tl can provide information about myocardial viability but not as reliably as PET. ECG, cardiac catheterization, and transthoracic echocardiography have no role in assessing myocardial viability.

23. D (Chapter 5)

Sentinel loop of bowel is a sign of localized inflammation and is associated with pancreatitis if it is found in the upper abdomen. The elevated alcohol level supports the diagnosis.

24. D (Chapter 8)

Ulnar deviation of the phalanges is classically associated with rheumatoid arthritis. The periarticular erosions may be seen in other conditions such as gout, but this is not the best answer given the rest of the information in the history.

25. B (Chapter 3)

The CT scan of the head shows a new high-attenuation left-sided subdural hematoma. It has the classic biconcave or crescent shape as opposed to an epidural, which has a biconvex, or lens, shape. There is also a chronic right-sided subdural hematoma, or hygroma as it is also called, when the blood products are replaced by CSF. A subarachnoid hemorrhage would have high-attenuation blood outlining the gyri or in the ventricles. Lymphoma and metastases appear as a mass or multiple masses in the brain parenchyma.

26. A (Chapter 9)

The most likely diagnosis from the history is a foreign-body aspiration, from a small piece of food. Most commonly, the food is a pea, a piece of corn, or a small nut. The right lung is more commonly affected, likely because the right mainstem bronchus comes off from the carina at a less acute angle than the left. Hyperinflation is the classic radiographic finding on CXR because the obstruction causes air trapping in the affected lung. Decubitus films will help to prove the diagnosis because the lung with the obstruction remains fully inflated even when it is the dependent side on the decubitus film.

27. C (Chapter 6)

The history is suspicious for a ureteral stone. In the acute setting, a noncontrast CT of the abdomen and pelvis (CT urogram) is the best test for diagnosing a ureteral calculus. An ultrasound may show secondary signs of ureteral obstruction, such as dilatation of the renal collecting system and proximal ureter, but it is not a good test for locating a ureteral stone. The IVP historically was the test of choice for the diagnosis of ureteral stones, but it has been replaced by the CT urogram, which is faster to perform and avoids the use of iodine-based IV contrast. A KUB may show calcifications but is not a specific test because pelvic phleboliths are common in many patients as well and may interfere with the diagnosis of a distal ureteral stone. MRI of the abdomen is useful for complicated renal masses, some of which may cause hematuria, but it is not used for suspected urolithiasis.

28. B (Chapter 2)

The history is consistent with a mass in the parotid gland, which narrows the differential to parotid carcinoma or pleo-morphic adenoma. The additional history of facial droop indicates invasion into the seventh cranial nerve, which only a malignant neoplasm would do. Therefore pleomorphic adenoma is excluded, leaving parotid carcinoma.

Mumps viral infection is uncommon because of vaccinations, would likely be associated with fever and malaise, and would not last for 3 months. A stroke would not have a facial mass, but it might present with a facial droop. A parapharyngeal abscess would also present more acutely and would have a different appearance, with a fluid collection in the more medially located parapharyngeal space.

29. D (Chapter 3)

The CT scan reveals multiple round, well-demarcated foci consistent with multiple metastases. Abscesses are not consistent with the history. Intracerebral hematomas would not appear so focal and well circumscribed. Multiple sclerosis does not usually have any findings on CT and can be seen only on MRI. Glioblastoma multiforme is commonly a large solitary, infiltrating lesion with surrounding edema.

30. B (Chapter 5)

The radiographs demonstrate a classic appearance of small-bowel obstruction with dilated loops of small bowel on the supine film and air-fluid levels on the upright film.

31. C (Chapter 4)

The CXR shows bilateral pleural cupping, left greater than right. Although this finding can be attributed to the superior rib fractures (note the arrows in Figure A-31), a CT scan of the chest should be obtained to identify a possible aortic injury that resulted in the hemothorax. If clinical suspicion for aortic injury exists, an aortogram can be performed. Although chest tubes are placed for hemothorax, a diagnosis is better

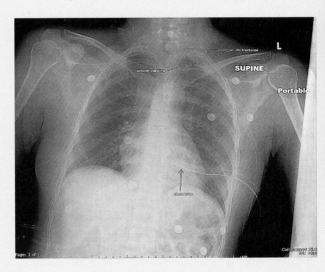

Figure A-31 • (Courtesy of University of Southern California Medical Center, Los Angeles, CA.)

obtained first. Surgical exploration is considered only when the clinical suspicion is very high and waiting for diagnostic studies would endanger the patient's life.

32. B (Chapter 9)

The upright film of the abdomen demonstrates a mass in the right upper abdomen, outlined by colonic gas (Figure A-32). This mass represents an intussusception located in the right colon. An intussusception can present as small bowel obstruction, but here no significantly distended small bowel segments are identified. Acute gastroenteritis usually presents with an increased volume of gas and some fluid within small and large bowel. Appendicitis can present with a mass (especially if a perforation has occurred) located in right lower quadrant. No extraluminal gas is seen on this film.

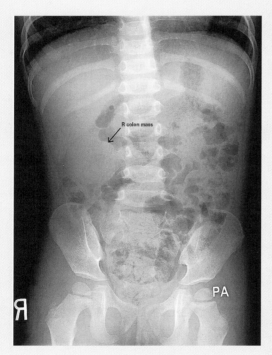

Figure A-32 • (Courtesy of University of Southern California Medical Center, Los Angeles, CA.)

33. B (Chapter 11)

Despite better results with CTPA, the radiation exposure to the patient is lower with a V/Q study and thus remains the preferred modality for evaluation of PE in pregnant patients.

34. D (Chapter 8)

Note the sunburst periosteal reaction within the proximal left tibia. This periosteal reaction is different from the "onion" layering of Ewing sarcoma. Chronic osteomyelitis may result in increased density of bone, but this periosteal reaction is exuberant. The joint, although it contains some osteoid deposition, does not demonstrate narrowing or erosion to suggest either rheumatoid or septic arthritis. No callus formation is present to suggest old fracture, and the extent of bone involvement is too large.

35. B (Chapter 6)

Circumferential urinary bladder wall thickening is most likely due to cystitis or bladder outlet obstruction by an enlarged prostate. Although carcinomatous involvement of the gland can cause enlargement, the best answer is B, as the prostate can be just hyperplastic. Transitional cell carcinoma of the urinary bladder usually causes an asymmetric mass. The conus medullaris syndrome presents with urinary retention and bowel incontinence. Metastatic disease to the urinary bladder, other than from the ureters, is rare.

36. A (Chapter 6)

The clinical history and the CT lead to the diagnosis of prostate carcinoma. Although the patient does not present with bone pain, bone metastases are very common and should be sought. Although whole-body rapid MRI sequence is sometimes mentioned, it is not a current practice. A follow-up CT scan of the abdomen and pelvis is often performed once therapy is instituted, and no mention of treatment is made in the text. Metastases to the lung from prostate carcinoma occur in advanced stages. If any clinical suspicion exists, a CT of the chest is preferred because lung metastases are not always conspicuous on a chest x-ray.

37. E (Chapter 4)

The CTPA demonstrates filling defects within the pulmonary arteries bilaterally (Figure A-37). No pneumothorax or aortic dissection is present. The ribs are intact. Bland (e.g., fibrin and

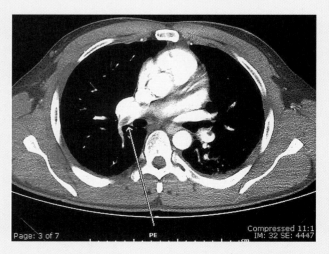

Figure A-37 • (Courtesy of University of Southern California Medical Center, Los Angeles, CA.)

platelets) and tumor emboli are seen usually lodged within the central pulmonary arteries. Septic PE commonly have a peripheral location and appearance of cavitary parenchymal nodules.

38. B (Chapter 11)

Risk stratification after MI is one of the four indications for stress cardiac scintigraphy, together with diagnosis of CAD, preoperative evaluation, and assessment of viable myocardium versus scar.

39. C (Chapter 4)

A CT of the chest is the best option to identify the underlying pathology for a recurrent or nonresolving pneumothorax. An MRI of the chest is not as sensitive for evaluating the lung parenchyma because of cardiac pulsation and breathing artifacts. A spontaneous pneumothorax may occur secondary to rupture of a pulmonary bleb (pneumatocele, bulla) or as the result of pleural metastasis. Idiopathic spontaneous pneumothorax has been documented in tall, thin young males. Osteosarcoma may present in young patients with a spontaneous pneumothorax due to lung metastases. A rib series may be obtained if there is suspicion that the patient has suffered trauma. An echocardiogram has no indication.

40. C (Chapter 2)

A non-contrast CT is the best option to evaluate the sinuses and the extent of sinusitis. If any neurologic deficits are present, an MRI of the brain is indicated to identify any brain abscesses. A skull scintigraphy has decreased spatial resolution (insufficient for evaluation of the sinuses), but would be helpful for diagnosing osteomyelitis. Plain films were the standard of care in the past. Ultrasound of the sinuses is not a performed examination.

41. B (Chapter 3)

Evaluation of the brain for primary or metastatic neoplasms is done by MRI with gadolinium (some lesions may not be appreciated before contrast administration). A CT with contrast may be obtained if the patient is unstable (i.e., cannot be in the MRI scanner for prolonged period) or if there are contraindications to undergo MRI (claustrophobia, pacemaker, cochlear implants), but not all brain lesions will be visualized. CT without contrast will demonstrate areas of hemorrhage, but it is suboptimal for detecting other than large lesions. A whole-body bone scan would be indicated in this setting to detect any bone metastases, but scintigraphy is not used for detecting brain lesions. Skull x-rays may sometimes be used to look for skull metastases.

42. E (Chapter 7)

At the mentioned beta-hCG level, a fetal pole should be identified. An ectopic pregnancy cannot be excluded based on imaging alone (not all ectopic pregnancies are visualized by ultrasound). A complete abortion may have occurred so that a pregnancy cannot be identified, but an ectopic should be still considered. The patient should be admitted and followed up with serial beta-hCG levels. A CT is not the imaging of choice to evaluate the female pelvis.

43. C (Chapter 5)

The image presented demonstrates an echogenic/bright curvilinear stone near the gallbladder neck with acoustic shadowing (echolucent/dark shadow in lower part of the image). The gallbladder wall thickness is measured with cursors at 0.73 cm (normal is 3 mm). If the clinical picture corresponds (elevated WBC, fevers), acute cholecystitis is diagnosed.

44. D (Chapter 1)

The first-line, least invasive, least time-consuming, and most easily obtainable test for suspected portal vein thrombosis is Doppler ultrasound. A gray scale ultrasound is used to evalute liver parenchyma. A CT of the abdomen with IV contrast is an alternative, but iodinated contrast allergic reactions and risk of iatrogenic renal insufficiency make this study less desirable. An MRI can be obtained but should not be used as a first line for the above indication.

45. D (Chapter 9)

A plain film of the abdomen, upright or cross-table lateral (if the infant cannot be held upright), is first obtained to evaluate for possible pneumoperitoneum and to identify the site of suspected intussusception. If the plain film fails to reveal an intussusception, an attempt at identifying it can be made with ultrasound. Although CT is a good modality, exposure to relatively high-level radiation is best avoided. MRI is not a good modality for evaluating bowel. A chest x-ray may show free air under the diaphragm but would not locate the intussusception.

46. C (Chapter 11)

External radiation was used in the past to treat Hodgkin disease, acne, tinea capitis, enlarged tonsils, and adenoids. It was strongly associated with a higher incidence of thyroid cancer. Age, sex, and diet have not been proven to be risk factors for thyroid cancer.

47. D (Chapter 11)

The current recommended approach for treatment of papillary thyroid cancer is surgical excision followed by ablation of residual thyroid tissue with ^{131}I. The patient is then followed up with whole-body diagnostic ^{123}I scans and measurement of thyroglobulin levels. Therefore the other answers are not correct.

ANSWERS

48. A (Chapter 1)

If esophageal injury is suspected, an esophagogram is recommended for diagnosis as soon as possible to prevent severe mediastinal infection. If the risk of aspiration is low (i.e., the patient is not obtunded or the airway is protected), Gastrografin is the preferred oral contrast agent because it does not cause mediastinitis if it extravasates through an esophageal laceration. Inhaled Gastrografin leads to pneumonitis. Barium is used in esophagograms in which an esophageal leak is not expected because its extravasation causes mediastinitis.

49. D (Chapter 8)

A 50% bone destruction has to occur before plain radiographs demonstrate any bone abnormality. If the clinical scenario indicates osteomyelitis, an MRI or bone scan of the area has to be obtained. Follow-up with repeat plain films would lead to a delay in diagnosis. A long course of IV antibiotics must be started for osteomyelitis. Amputation is usually planned if the osteomyelitis is extensive or if the patient does not respond to medical treatment.

50. D. (Chapter 11)

The GI bleeding scan is the most sensitive procedure used for detection of lower GI bleeds. It is used for identification of the location of a bleed before angiography. CT scan of the abdomen and abdominal x-rays are not valuable in the assessment of a GI bleed.

51. E (Chapter 4)

The CXR demonstrates a chest tube over the right chest wall. A horizontal air-fluid level on an upright CXR should signal that both fluid and gas are present within the pleural space. The fluid may be a simple pleural effusion or blood (in the setting of trauma). Sometimes a hemothorax may be the result of a traumatic chest tube placement. The mediastinum is not widened to suggest large vessel injury.

52. C (Chapter 9)

The study is a VCUG demonstrating contrast reflux into the renal calices during micturition. The urethra is of normal caliber. If ureteral obstruction were to be present, the contrast would not have flown retrograde past the obstruction point, and the renal ultrasound should have shown hydronephrosis.

53. E (Chapter 7)

The cursors outline an ectopic pregnancy. A dilated fallopian tube usually has low echogenicity and a tubular configuration. No intrauterine pregnancy is imaged. Given the patient's positive pregnancy test, an ovarian neoplasm is unlikely. An appendix located in the left lower quadrant is a rare occurrence.

54. B (Chapter 4)

The film shows a right upper lobe infiltrate and blunting of the right costophrenic angle. With the short history of fevers and cough, pneumonia with associated pleural effusion is the most likely diagnosis. It is very important to order a delayed follow-up film to make sure the pneumonia has resolved and is not masking a malignancy. A lobe collapse would result in volume loss with mediastinal shift toward the affected side and elevation of the minor fissure. A lung contusion could have this appearance, but no trauma is mentioned in the history. No artifact is present on this film.

55. A (Chapter 7)

This picture depicts a classic image of a midcycle ovary just before rupture of the dominant follicle and release of the ovum. A simple cyst without a thickened wall, septations, or internal echoes in a woman of reproductive age is highly suggestive of a benign process. This patient should be reassured that this is a normal physiologic finding. Simple cysts larger than 3.5 cm should be followed up for resolution in 1 or 2 months.

56. D (Chapter 5)

Lucency is seen under both diaphragms and represents extraluminal gas (pneumoperitoneum), a surgical emergency. In this case a perforated ulcer should be sought for as the cause.

57. B (Chapter 7)

Single or multiple solid circular masses adjacent to or inside of the uterus on ultrasound are most suggestive of fibroids. Fibroids are common benign pelvic masses consisting of smooth muscle. They are commonly asymptomatic but may be associated with pain, bleeding, or infertility problems, depending on their size and location. Fibroids can be submucosal, intramural, or subserosal. Management options are dictated by symptoms and range from annual follow-up to removal of the entire uterus (hysterectomy).

58. C (Chapter 6)

The image shows two simple right renal cysts that do not require follow-up or confirmation by other imaging modality. A urology consult is obtained in complex cysts or masses suspicious for malignancy because the patient may require partial or total nephrectomy. The patient should be reassured that simple cysts are a benign finding.

59. B (Chapter 5)

The CT image obtained without IV contrast because of the patient's renal insufficiency (refer to Chapter 1 for creatinine levels and approach before a contrast study can be obtained) shows inflammatory changes in and around the pancreas. An ultrasound to evaluate for choledocholithiasis is indicated.

Note the low density of the liver (lower than the kidney and abdominal wall muscles) representing fatty liver. The duodenum contains oral contrast. Only if imaging difficulty is encountered at the easily accessible ultrasound (i.e., bowel gas obscures the common bile duct) should magnetic resonance cholangiopancreatography (MRCP) be obtained. A nuclear scintigraphy scan (HIDA), described in Chapter 11, is used for diagnosing acute cholecystitis. Only 20% of gallstones are radio-opaque, so a KUB is occasionally diagnostic.

60. E (Chapter 3)

The sagittal image from a gadolinium-enhanced T1-weighted sequence MRI (the CSF is dark and the scalp fat is white) shows an enhancing mass within the fourth ventricle (astrocytoma). A cyst or fourth ventricular enlargement should appear dark (low signal intensity), the same as the CSF.

61. D (Chapter 4)

The CXR demonstrates an enlarged cardiac silhouette and interstitial edema. The right midlung linear horizontal density represents a small volume of fluid in the minor fissure. No pneumothorax, large pleural effusions, or rib fractures are present.

62. A (Chapter 3)

The image shows dilated third and lateral ventricles (Figure A-62). Looking at the brain surface, the cerebral sulci are normal in size (not deep). Enlarged ventricles accompanied by deepened cerebral sulci resulting from volume loss (cerebral atrophy)

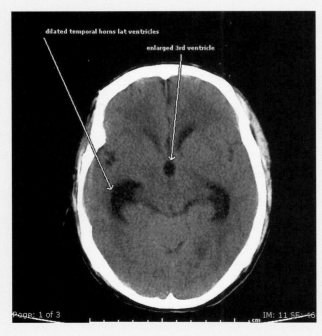

Figure A-62 • (Courtesy of University of Southern California Medical Center, Los Angeles, CA.)

are commonly seen in older patients and are of no clinical concern.

63. B (Chapter 3)

A cause for the ventricular dilatation has to be sought (such as a metastasis obstructing the sylvian acqueduct or a mass within the fourth ventricle); so an MRI of the brain with gadolinium needs to be ordered. If the patient suffered a traumatic hemorrhage, it should be evident on this initial scan. A skull fracture in a plane parallel to the image can be missed by CT, so a plain skull film is sometimes ordered. An ischemic stroke may not be evident on CT even for 24 hours, after which a low density (dark) area should be visualized. If suspicion of recent stroke (less than 3 hours) exists, an emergent MRI should be obtained before thrombolytic therapy is begun. CT provides less anatomic detail. The MRI can detect restriction of water diffusion in the area of ischemia before the infarction occurs (when CT would become positive).

64. D (Chapter 5)

The arrows point to strictured segments of ileum due to Crohn enteritis (ileitis). The lesions occur in nonadjacent segments of bowel ("skip lesions"). No abdominal mass is evident. In bowel obstruction, multiple small-bowel segments would be distended. Parasitic infestation would show as filling defects within the bowel lumen (in cases in which the parasites are large enough, such as *Ascaris lumbricoides,* 8 to 12 inches long) and eventually bowel obstruction.

65. E (Chapter 4)

The CXR (Figure A-65) shows the endotracheal tip too deep, into the right mainstem bronchus, resulting in left lung collapse. The right-sided heart border is not seen because the

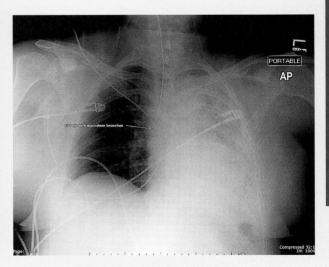

Figure A-65 • (Courtesy of University of Southern California Medical Center, Los Angeles, CA.)

mediastinum is shifted leftward. If the left hemithorax opacification were due to a large pleural effusion, the mediastinum would have shifted rightward. At times the mediastinum does not shift if there is a combination of pleural effusion and atelectasis (volume loss) on the same side of the chest.

66. A (Chapter 11)

V/Q scintigraphy demonstrates a lack of peripheral perfusion that is not matched by the ventilation portion of the study. The study is then read as high probability for pulmonary emboli. In asthma, some air trapping may be present, and the inhaled radionuclide will clear slowly from the affected lung segments. In this study the ventilation is homogeneous. If several metallic objects overlie the patient during the study, the gamma camera would not detect radiation from the particular lung regions. The technicians are usually diligent about removing any artifact-causing devices.

67. A (Chapter 11)

Given the findings compatible with multiple PE, the patient should be treated.

68. C (Chapter 10)

The lumen of the aorta is opacified with contrast, but within its wall a mural thrombus is present (low density/attenuation at periphery) (Figure A-68). The small curvilinear densities at the periphery of the aorta represent mural calcifications of atherosclerotic vascular disease. The IVC is also labeled.

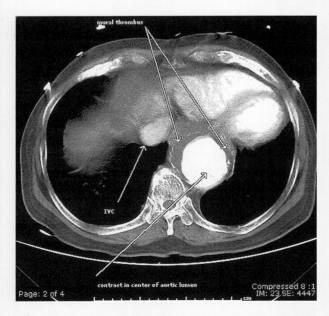

Figure A-68 • (Courtesy of University of Southern California Medical Center, Los Angeles, CA.)

69. C (Chapter 10)

The patient needs a surgical evaluation for repair of this large thoracoabdominal aneurysm (synthetic graft). The larger the aneurysm (the cutoff number for the diameter is 5 cm), the higher the likelihood of rupture. The patient requires evaluation of coronary arteries before surgery because the aneurysms have a high association with atherosclerotic vascular disease.

70. D (Chapter 8)

The best imaging for suspected multiple myeloma is a metastatic skeletal survey (skull, spine, femurs, humeri, and pelvis). The punched-out lesions are characteristic. Of course, the laboratory workup is confirmatory. The bone lesions of multiple myeloma do not take up the radioactive tracer used for bone scans, so this test would be wrong. MRI of the spine is indicated only if cord compression is suspected. A CT scan of the spine is not commonly performed other than in the setting of trauma.

71. D (Chapter 10)

If a DVT extends to the level of the IVC, an IVC filter should be placed in the suprarenal IVC.

72. C (Chapter 10)

Nephrostomy tubes should ideally be placed in a posterior calyx because this is the best approach to avoid injury to renal vasculature.

73. B (Chapter 10)

Before any interventional radiology procedure, it is important to confirm PT, PTT, INR, and platelets to evaluate for any coagulopathy. BUN, and creatinine if contrast is going to be administered. As this patient is known to have biliary obstruction, bilirubin levels, although important, will not directly affect whether the procedure will be performed or not.

74. D (Chapter 10)

Posttraumatic pseudoaneuryms most commonly occur at the level of the ligamentum arteriosum, at least those that survive the trip to the hospital. Transections of the ascending aorta are almost uniformly fatal and usually are not seen in a hospital setting.

75. E (Chapter 10)

The clinical triad of buttock claudication, impotence, and decreased femoral pulses is called Leriche syndrome and is secondary to atherosclerotic aortoiliac occlusive disease. The other diseases do not cause this clinical triad.

Appendix: Evidence-Based Resources

Chapter 1

Di Carli MF. Advances in positron emission tomography. J Nucl Cardiol 2004;11:719–732.

Garcia-Ruiz C, Martinez-Vea A, Sempere T, et al. Low risk of contrast nephropathy in high-risk patients undergoing spiral computed tomography angiography with the contrast medium iopromide and prophylactic oral hydratation. Clin Nephrol 2004;61:170–176.

Radhakrishnan S, Manoharan S, Fleet M. Repeat survey of current practice regarding corticosteroid prophylaxis for patients at increased risk of adverse reaction to intravascular contrast agents. Clin Radiol 2005;60:58–63.

Rashid ST, Salman M, Myint F, et al. Prevention of contrast-induced nephropathy in vascular patients undergoing angiography: a randomized controlled trial of intravenous N-acetylcysteine. J Vasc Surg 2004;40:1136–1141.

Chapter 2

Arrington JA. Imaging of the upper airway and sinuses. Clin Allergy Immunol 2000;15:263–286.

Henrot P, Blum A, Toussaint B, et al. Dynamic maneuvers in local staging of head and neck malignancies with current imaging techniques: principles and clinical applications. Radiographics 2003;23:1201–1213.

Mack MG, Balzer JO, Herzog C, Vogl TJ. Multi-detector CT: head and neck imaging. Eur Radiol 2003;13(suppl)5:M121–M126.

Chapter 3

Calfee DP, Wispelwey B. Brain abscess. Semin Neurol 2000;20:353–360.

Castillo M, Mukherji SK. Diffusion-weighted imaging in the evaluation of intracranial lesions. Semin Ultrasound CT MR 2000;21:405–416.

Provenzale JM, Jahan R, Naidich TP, Fox AJ. Assessment of the patient with hyperacute stroke: imaging and therapy. Radiology 2003;229:347–359.

Pueschel JK, Ashby LS, Shapiro WR. Brain tumors. Cancer Chemother Biol Response Modif 2003;21:655–681.

Romano A, Bozzao A, Bonamini M, et al. Diffusion-weighted MR imaging: clinical applications in neuroradiology. Radiol Med 2003;106:521–548.

Sano T, Horiguchi H. Von Hippel-Lindau disease. Microsc Res Tech 2003;60:159–164.

Schellinger PD. MRI-guided therapy in acute stroke. Expert Rev Cardiovasc Ther 2003;1:569–580.

Spence AM, Mankoff DA, Muzi M. Positron emission tomography imaging of brain tumors. Neuroimaging Clin N Am 2003;13:717–739.

Vogel H, Fuller GN. Primitive neuroectodermal tumors, embryonal tumors, and other small cell and poorly differentiated malignant neoplasms of the central and peripheral nervous systems. Ann Diagn Pathol 2003;7:387–398.

Chapter 4

Ball CG, Hameed SM, Evans D, et al. Canadian Trauma Trials Collaborative. Occult pneumothorax in the mechanically ventilated trauma patient. Can J Surg 2003;46:373–379.

Costello J, Hogg K. CT pulmonary angiogram compared with ventilation-perfusion scan for the diagnosis of pulmonary embolism in patients with cardiorespiratory disease. Emerg Med J 2003;20:547–548.

Gotway MB, Dawn SK. Thoracic aorta imaging with multislice CT. Radiol Clin N Am 2003;41:521–543.

Nijkeuter M, Huisman MV. The role of helical CT in the diagnosis of pulmonary embolism. Pathophysiol Haemost Thromb 2004;33:319–326.

Worsley DF, Alavi A. Radionuclide imaging of acute pulmonary embolism. Semin Nucl Med 2003;33:259–278.

Chapter 5

Bingener J, Schwesinger WH, Chopra S, et al. Does the correlation of acute cholecystitis on ultrasound and at surgery reflect a mirror image? Am J Surg 2004;188:703–707.

Frager D. Intestinal obstruction role of CT. Gastroenterol Clin N Am 2002;31:777–799.

Ziessman HA. Acute cholecystitis, biliary obstruction, and biliary leakage. Semin Nucl Med 2003;33:279–296.

Chapter 6
Purohit RS, Shinohara K, Meng MV, Carroll PR. Imaging clinically localized prostate cancer. Urol Clin North Am. 2003 May;30(2):279–293.

Schreyer HH, Uggowitzer MM, Ruppert-Kohlmayr A. Helical CT of the urinary organs. Eur Radiol 2002;12:575–591.

Xie Q, Zhang J, Wu PH, et al. Bladder transitional cell carcinoma: correlation of contrast enhancement on computed tomography with histological grade and tumour angiogenesis. Clin Radiol 2005;60:215–223.

Chapter 7
Davidson KG, Dubinsky TJ. Ultrasonographic evaluation of the endometrium in postmenopausal vaginal bleeding. Radiol Clin N Am 2003;41:769–780.

Dialani V, Levine D. Ectopic pregnancy: a review. Ultrasound Quart 2004;20:105–117.

Shagam JY. Ultrasound assessment of uterine disorders. Radiol Technol 2000;72:11–22.

Chapter 8
Furlow B. Radiography of bone tumors and lesions. Radiol Technol 2001;72:455–469.

Miller SL, Hoffer FA. Malignant and benign bone tumors. Radiol Clin North Am 2001;39:673–699.

Museru LM, Mcharo CN. Chronic osteomyelitis: a continuing orthopaedic challenge in developing countries. Int Orthop 2001;25:127–131.

Chapter 9
Byrne AT, Geoghegan T, Govender P, et al. The imaging of intussusception. Clin Radiol 2005;60:39–46.

Hansson S, Dhamey M, Sigstrom O, et al. Dimercapto-succinic acid scintigraphy instead of voiding cystourethrography for infants with urinary tract infection. J Urol 2004;72:1071–1073.

Hernandez JA, Swischuk LE, Angel CA. Validity of plain films in intussusception. Emerg Radiol 2004;10:323–326.

Chapter 10
Herborn CU, Goyen M, Quick HH, et al. Whole-body 3D MR angiography of patients with peripheral arterial occlusive disease. AJR Am J Roentgenol 2004;182:1427–1434.

Kaufman JA, Lee MJ. Vascular and Interventional Radiology: The Requisites. Philadelphia: Elsevier, 2004.

Kinney TB. Update on inferior vena cava filters. J Vasc Interv Radiol 2003;14:425–440.

Kuo WT, Lee DE, Saad WE, et al. Superselective microcoil embolization for the treatment of lower gastrointestinal hemorrhage. J Vasc Interv Radiol 2003;14:1503–1509.

Moore KL, Agur AM. Essential Clinical Anatomy. Baltimore: William & Wilkins, 1995.

Ofer A, Nitecki SS, Linn Shai, et al. Multidetector CT angiography of peripheral vascular disease: a prospective comparison with intraarterial digital subtraction angiography. AJR Am J Roentgenol 2003;180:719–724.

Razavi MK, Lee DS, Hofmann LV. Catheter-directed thrombolytic therapy for limb ischemia: current status and controversies. J Vasc Interv Radiol 2004;15:13–23.

Schenker MP, Duszak R, Soulen MC, et al. Upper gastrointestinal hemorrhage and transcatheter embolotherapy: clinical and technical factors impacting success and survival. J Vasc Interv Radiol 2001;12:1263–1271.

vanSonnenberg E, Mueller PR, Ferrucci JT. Percutaneous drainage of 250 abdominal abscesses and fluid collections. I. Results, failures and complications. Radiology 1984;151:337–341.

Won JY, Lee DY, Shim WH, et al. Elective endovascular treatment of descending thoracic aortic aneurysms and chronic dissections with stent-grafts. J Vasc Interv Radiol 2001;12: 575–582.

Zagoria RJ. Genitourinary Radiology: The Requisites. Philadelphia: Mosby, 2004.

Chapter 11
Alobaidi M, Gupta R, Jafri SZ, Fink-Bennet DM. Current trends in imaging evaluation of acute cholecystitis. Emerg Radiol 2004;10:256–258.

Cohen JB, Kalinyak JE, McDougall IR. Modern management of differentiated thyroid cancer. Cancer Biother Radiopharm 2003;18:689–705.

Delbeke D, Martin WH. Metabolic imaging with FDG: a primer. Cancer J 2004;10:201–13.

Hachamovitch R, Berman DS. New frontiers in risk stratification using stress myocardial perfusion single photon emission computed tomography. Curr Opin Cardiol 2003;18: 494–502.

Howarth DM, Tang K, Lees W. The clinical utility of nuclear medicine imaging for the detection of occult gastrointestinal haemorrhage. Nucl Med Commun 2002;23:591–594.

Massoud TF, Gambhir SS. Molecular imaging in living subjects: seeing fundamental biological processes in a new light. Genes Dev 2003;17:545–580.

Savelli G, Maffioli L, Maccauro M, et al. Bone scintigraphy and the added value of SPECT (single photon emission tomography) in detecting skeletal lesions. Q J Nucl Med 2001;45: 27–37.

Index

NOTES

NOTES

NOTES

NOTES

NOTES

NOTES

NOTES

NOTES

NOTES

NOTES